theclinics.com

Robert A. Smith, DVM, MS
CONSULTING EDITOR

VETERINARY CLINICS OF NORTH AMERICA

Food Animal Practice

Ruminant Parasitology

GUEST EDITOR
Lora Rickard Ballweber, MS, DVM

November 2006 • Volume 22 • Number 3

SAUNDERS
An Imprint of Elsevier, Inc.
PHILADELPHIA LONDON TORONTO MONTREAL SYDNEY TOKYO

W.B. SAUNDERS COMPANY
A Division of Elsevier Inc.

Elsevier, Inc., 1600 John F. Kennedy Blvd., Suite 1800, Philadelphia, PA 19103-2899

http://www.vetfood.theclinics.com

VETERINARY CLINICS OF NORTH AMERICA: FOOD ANIMAL PRACTICE
November 2006
Editor: John Vassallo; j.vassallo@elsevier.com

Volume 22, Number 3
ISSN 0749-0720
ISBN 1-4160-3826-4

Veterinary Clinics of North America: Food Animal Practice (ISSN 0749-0720) is published in March, July, and November by W.B. Saunders, 360 Park Avenue South, New York, NY 10010-1710. Business and Editorial Offices: 1600 John F. Kennedy Blvd., Suite 1800, Philadelphia, PA 19103-2899. Accounting and Circulation Offices: 6277 Sea Harbor Drive, Orlando, FL 32887-4800. Periodicals postage paid at New York, NY and additional mailing offices. Subscription prices are $132.00 per year for US individuals, $211.00 per year for US institutions, $66.00 per year for US students and residents, $154.00 per year for Canadian individuals, $270.00 per year for Canadian institutions, $182.00 per year for international individuals, $270.00 per year for international institutions and $94.00 per year for Canadian and foreign students/residents. To receive student/resident rate, orders must be accompained by name of affiliated institution, date of term, and the *signature* of program/residency coordinator on institution letterhead. Orders will be billed at individual rate until proof of status is received. Foreign air speed delivery is included in all *Clinics* subscription prices. All prices are subject to change without notice. **POSTMASTER**: Send address changes to *Veterinary Clinics of North America: Food Animal Practice*, Elsevier Periodicals Customer Service, 6277 Sea Harbor Drive, Orlando, FL 32887-4800, USA; phone: (+1) (877) 839-7126 [toll free number for US customers], or (+1) (407) 345-4020 [customers outside US]; fax: (+1) (407) 363-1354; e-mail: usjcs@elsevier.com.

Reprints. For copies of 100 or more, of articles in this publication, please contact the Commercial Reprints Department, Elsevier Inc., 360 Park Avenue South, New York, New York 10010-1710. Tel.: (212) 633-3813; Fax: (212) 462-1935; e-mail: Reprints@elsevier.com.

Veterinary Clinics of North America: Food Animal Practice is covered in *Current Contents/Agriculture, Biology and Environmental Sciences, Index Medicus, and Excerpta Medica.*

Printed in the United States of America.

CONSULTING EDITOR

ROBERT A. SMITH, DVM, MS, Diplomate, American Board of Veterinary Practitioners; Veterinary Research and Consulting Services, LLC, Stillwater, Oklahoma

GUEST EDITOR

LORA RICKARD BALLWEBER, MS, DVM, Diplomate, European Veterinary Parasitology College; Associate Professor, Clinical Parasitology, Department of Microbiology, Immunology and Pathology, Colorado State University, Ft. Collins, Colorado

CONTRIBUTORS

LORA RICKARD BALLWEBER, MS, DVM, Diplomate, European Veterinary Parasitology College; Associate Professor, Clinical Parasitology, Department of Microbiology, Immunology and Pathology, Colorado State University, Ft. Collins, Colorado

KATHERINE D. BARDSLEY, MSc, Manager of Diagnostic Parasitology and Clinical Pathology Sections of the Wyoming State Veterinary Laboratory, Laramie, Wyoming

ROBERTO CORTINAS, DVM, Senior Scientist, Department of Veterinary and Biomedical Sciences, University of Minnesota, St. Paul, Minnesota

THOMAS M. CRAIG, DVM, PhD, Professor, Department of Veterinary Pathobiology, Texas A&M University, College Station, Texas

JOHN E. CREWS, DVM, MS, Diagnostic Veterinary Manager, Florida Department of Agriculture and Consumer Services, State of Florida, Fort Meade, Florida

J. P. DUBEY, MVSc, PhD, Senior Scientist, United States Department of Agriculture, Agricultural Research Service, Animal and Natural Resources Institute, Beltsville Agricultural Research Center, Beltsville, Maryland

LOUIS C. GASBARRE, PhD, Research Leader, Bovine Functional Genomics Laboratory, Agricultural Research Service, United Sates Department of Agriculture, Beltsville, Maryland

WILLIAM R. JOLLEY, MSc, PhD, Associate Professor, Department of Veterinary Sciences, University of Wyoming; Supervisor of Diagnostic Parasitology and Clinical Pathology Sections of the Wyoming State Veterinary Laboratory, Laramie, Wyoming

CARL J. JONES, PhD, Professor and Head, Department of Entomology and Plant Pathology, University of Tennessee, Knoxville, Tennessee

DAVID S. LINDSAY, PhD, Professor, Department of Biomedical Sciences and Pathobiology, Virginia-Maryland Regional College of Veterinary Medicine, Virginia Tech, Blacksburg, Virginia

RYAN M. O'HANDLEY, BSc, PhD, Senior Research Fellow, Environmental Biotechnology Cooperative Research Centre, School of Veterinary and Biomedical Sciences, Murdoch University, Perth, Australia; Adjunct Professor, Department of Health Management, Atlantic Veterinary College, Charlottetown, Prince Edward Island, Canada

MERLE E. OLSON, DVM, MSc, President, Bow Valley Research, Calgary; Research Director, MBEC Bioproducts, University of Calgary, Calgary; Adjunct Professor, BioMedical Engineering, University of Alberta, Edmonton, Alberta, Canada

CARLA PANUSKA, MS, PhD, Assistant Research Professor, College of Veterinary Medicine, Mississippi State University, Mississippi State, Mississippi

D. OWEN RAE, DVM, MPVM, Associate Professor of Veterinary Medicine, Food Animal Reproduction and Medicine Service, Veterinary Medical Center, College of Veterinary Medicine, University of Florida, Gainesville, Florida

BERT E. STROMBERG, PhD, Professor of Parasitology and Associate Dean for Research and Graduate Programs, College of Veterinary Medicine, University of Minnesota, St. Paul, Minnesota

Chris A. TUCKER, PhD, Department of Animal Sciences, University of Arkansas, Fayetteville, Arkansas

THOMAS A. YAZWINSKI, PhD, Department of Animal Sciences, University of Arkansas, Fayetteville, Arkansas

ANNE M. ZAJAC, DVM, PhD, Associate Professor, Department of Biomedical Sciences and Pathobiology, Virginia-Maryland Regional College of Veterinary Medicine, Virginia Tech, Blacksburg, Virginia

CONTENTS

FORTHCOMING ISSUES

March 2007

Cow/Calf Nutrition
Larry C. Hollis, DVM, M Ag
K.C. Olson, PhD, *Guest Editors*

July 2007

Beef Cattle Nutrition
Larry C. Hollis, DVM, M Ag
K.C. Olson, PhD, *Guest Editors*

November 2007

Diagnostics
Robert J. Callan, DVM, PhD, *Guest Editor*

RECENT ISSUES

July 2006

Stocker Cattle Management
Mark F. Spire, DVM, MS
Robert A. Smith, DVM, MS, *Guest Editors*

March 2006

Barnyard Epidemiology and Performance Assessment
Pamela L. Ruegg, DVM, MPVM, *Guest Editor*

November 2005

Emergency Medicine and Critical Care of Cattle
Sheila M. McGuirk, DMV, PhD, and
Simon F. Peek, BVSc, MRCVS, PhD
Guest Editors

ELSEVIER
SAUNDERS

Vet Clin Food Anim
22 (2006) xi–xii

VETERINARY
CLINICS
Food Animal Practice

Preface

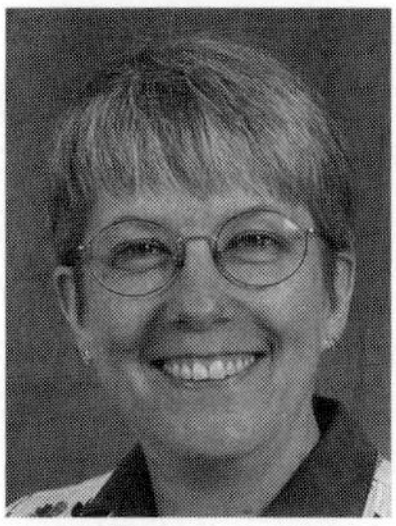

Lora Rickard Ballweber, MS, DVM
Guest Editor

Approximately 20 years ago, the American Association of Veterinary Parasitologists sponsored an issue of the *Veterinary Clinics of North America: Food Animal Practice*. The issue, edited by Drs. R. P. Herd, H. C. Gibbs, and K. D. Murrell, was entitled "Parasites: Epidemiology and Control" and soon became the standard reference on the epidemiology and control of both ecto- and endoparasites in ruminants and swine. However, much has happened in the intervening years, and it was considered time for an update. When approached, I was thrilled to lead this effort and have learned much. For example, many issues from 20 years ago are still around, the most obvious of which is anthelmintic resistance. What's more, understanding of the basic epidemiology of the gastrointestinal nematodes, to a great extent, comes from information derived from studies conducted 15 to 20 years ago. Whether the repeated use of anthelmintics over this timeframe, changes in management practices, climatic change, or other unidentified processes have altered those patterns has not really been investigated. On the other hand, new ways of looking at this same information have resulted in the exploration of novel parasiticides and fresh approaches to combating anthelmintic resistance. In contrast to the nematodes, great strides have been made in our understanding of other parasitic diseases, some of which we knew little, if anything, about 20 years ago. Most prominent here are many of the protozoal parasites, as evidenced by the increased article length compared with the 1986 edition.

doi:10.1016/j.cvfa.2006.08.002

The most important (re)observation I made was how generous the people are with whom we work. I wish to thank all of the authors who contributed their time and energy so that this issue could be produced, many of whom did so despite more pressing worries and I am in their debt. Unfortunately, not all topics from the previous issue could be included in the update. Missing are the swine chapters and information on ruminant trematodes and cestodes. Despite these shortcomings, the hope is that this issue, in the words of Drs. Herd, Gibbs, and Murrell, "... will introduce new concepts to those not yet exposed to them, dispel many old myths, and challenge young research workers to fill in important gaps in our knowledge" [1].

Lora Rickard Ballweber, MS, DVM
Department of Microbiology, Immunology and Pathology
1619 Campus Delivery
Colorado State University
Ft. Collins, CO 80523-1619, USA

E-mail address: lora.ballweber@colostate.edu

Reference

[1] Herd RP, Gibbs HC, Murrell KD. Foreword. Vet Clin North Am Food Anim Pract 1986;2: 203.

ELSEVIER
SAUNDERS

Vet Clin Food Anim
22 (2006) 501–527

VETERINARY
CLINICS
Food Animal Practice

A Sampling of Factors Relative to the Epidemiology of Gastrointestinal Nematode Parasites of Cattle in the United States

Thomas A. Yazwinski, PhD*, Chris A. Tucker, PhD

Department of Animal Sciences, B110D Animal Science, University of Arkansas, Fayetteville, AR 72701, USA

Gastrointestinal (GI) nematodosis of cattle is a parasitic condition resulting from an immense and seemingly forever-expanding array of factors. Countless determinants influence the incidence and severity of the species-specific infections that occur in cattle, determinants that affect the free-living or environmental stages of the parasites and the parasitic stages. Excellent reviews of epidemiological cycles engaged by the many cattle nematodes have been published, and the reader is advised to access these for a more thorough recount of the prominent and obscure nematodes that populate cattle and their pastures [1–3]. A commonality runs through the life histories of the GI cattle nematodes with only a few exceptions. As a group, they are oviparous, with separate sexes and direct life cycles, proceeding through four molts and six stages divided between the host and the environment. This seemingly simple progression, however, is influenced to a varying degree by hundreds of factors, ultimately resulting in parasitisms that vary region to region, farm to farm, pasture to pasture, season to season, and host to host. The multiple species infections that are the norm in cattle vary in detriment to the host from miniscule to acute. The vast majority of animals have a subclinical or economic level of parasitism undetectable to the eye but quantified more accurately by treatment-induced improved performance (eg, feed efficiency, nitrogen balance, weight gain, milk production). Unfortunately, the results of treatment (effectiveness and improved animal performance) sometimes can be as varied as the parasitisms that are being treated.

* Corresponding author.
E-mail address: yazwinsk@uark.edu (T.A. Yazwinski).

doi:10.1016/j.cvfa.2006.07.005

Given the diverse nature of GI nematodosis and the varied responses that result from treatment relative to effectiveness and animal performance, one can appreciate the room for controversies, both long standing and recently evolved, that perfuse the interpretations and viewpoints integral to GI nematode epidemiology. The actual life histories of the nematodes themselves have been, for the most part, a matter of observation and documentation. The long-standing controversies involve the sustainability of parasite controls [4], the extent to which controls should be used [5], and which control measures (chemical and nonchemical) should be developed or used [6]. A more recent controversy involves the magnitude and spectrum of resistance among the macrocyclic lactones [7]. Drug resistance is an important element in GI nematode epidemiology, and it is in this regard that it is discussed briefly in this article.

The nematodes

A list of the nematodes isolated from domesticated cattle (*Bos taurus* and *B indicus*) in the United States is presented in Table 1 [8–10]. Also provided for most nematode species listed are prepotence factors, characteristics displayed or used by the nematodes that have been observed as contributing to their success. Of the 26 listed species, 10 are considered the most significant because of their extensive prevalence and veterinary importance and are discussed briefly.

Haemonchus placei and *H contortus* (the latter more extensively involved than was previously believed [11]) are the "barber pole", large stomach, twisted stomach, or wire worms of cattle. Resident in the abomasum, they follow the trichostrongyle life cycle, are highly hematophagic, exhibit some degree of seasonal inhibition and periparturient rise, and for the most part are restricted to the south and southeast United States as major cattle parasites. Extensive genomes (nuclear and mitochondrial), capacity for genotypic adaptation to elements of selection (eg, nematocides), long generation time, and high fecundities are attributes that have allowed *Haemonchus* to plague sheep production around the world and now account for their emerging importance in the United States cattle industry [11,12].

Ostertagia ostertagi is the brown or medium stomach worm, and is recognized as the most important nematode parasite of cattle raised in temperate climates. This nematode uses the trichostrongyle life cycle and is resident in the abomasum. Singular in cattle is this worm's ability to developmentally arrest (seasonal and intraburden) and evade effective immune regulation by the host [13]. Northern and southern patterns of seasonal arrestment are well established in the Unite States [14], with *Ostertagia* spanning adverse weather conditions in mucosal nodules as inhibited early fourth-stage larvae (IEL_4). In a set of studies [15], it was shown that when northern and southern strains were moved to the opposite geographic tier, the original timing of inhibition was generally lost within 2 years, but the geographically correct inhibition patterns were not correspondingly adopted.

Table 1
Gastrointestinal nematode parasites of domestic cattle in North America

Genus	Species	Prepotence factor
Haemonchus	*placei*[a]	Extensive genome, resistance, inhibition, long patencies
	contortus[a]	Extensive genome, resistance, inhibition, long patencies
	similis[c]	—
Ostertagia	*ostertagi*[a]	Seasonal inhibition, immunity evasion
	bisonis[c]	—
	leptospicularis[c]	—
Trichostrongylus	*axei*[a]	No host age limitation
Cooperia	*oncophora*[a]	ML tolerance
	punctata[a]	ML tolerance
	pectinata[a]	ML tolerance
	surnabada[a]	ML tolerance
	curticei[c]	—
	spatulata[b]	—
Nematodirus	*helvetianus*[a]	Environmental resistance
	filicollis[c]	Environmental resistance
	spathiger[b]	Environmental resistance
Trichostrongylus	*colubriformis*[b]	Sheep reservoir
	longispicularis[c]	Sheep reservoir
Strongyloides	*papillosus*[a]	Heterogonic and homogonic
Capillaria	*bovis*[c]	—
Bunostomum	*phlebotomum*[b]	Skin or oral infection routes Long patencies
Toxocara	*vitulorum*[c]	—
Chabertia	*ovina*[c]	—
Oesophagostomum	*radiatum*[a]	Skin or oral infection routes
	venulosum[c]	—
Trichuris	*ovis*[b]	Environmental resistance

[a] Significant prevalence and veterinary importance.
[b] Limited incidence.
[c] Only rarely observed.

Trichostrongylus axei is the small or minute stomach worm. It follows the trichostrongyle life cycle with no tendency for predictable arrestment at any developmental stage. It is of restricted prevalence (present in <10% of individual animal coprocultures from most farms), but is not restricted in incidence by animal age or prior exposure. *T axei* perhaps enjoys a shroud of protection from effective immune responses from co-infecting *Ostertagia*. *T axei* usually is present in low numbers, but has been found in populations that rival those of adult *Ostertagia* in yearlings [16] and in adult cows [17].

Several *Cooperia* species infect cattle in the United States with *C oncophora*, *C punctata*, and *C pectinata* being the most prevalent. They follow the trichostrongyle life cycle and reside in the proximal small intestine. Significant burdens are restricted to animals 3 years of age or younger. No tendencies for predictable developmental arrestment have been documented, but sizable populations of fourth-stage larvae under apparent inhibition have been observed, resulting from intraburden inhibition [18] or continuous, low-level, non-efficacious avermectin usage (Yazwinski, unpublished data). The cooperiads have long been considered worthy of only measured consideration because of their low degree of pathogenicity relative to other nematodes and the fact that they are immunologically controlled by the end of an animal's second grazing season. At present, however, they are receiving far greater attention because of their resistance to the macrocyclic lactones [19,20] and observations that resistance may be linked to greater pathogenicity [21]. The associative nature of resistance and pathogenicity may be nothing more than a random coselection of genotypes. Alternatively, because the effect of macrocyclic lactones is cumulative over distinct neuromuscular compartments of susceptible nematodes, strains with expanded neural or muscular capacity would be inherently more resistant and at the same time more pathogenically active (eg, pharyngeal feeding, thigmokinetic activity).

Nematodirus helvetianus is the thread-necked worm of the small intestine, and uses the trichostrongyle life cycle with a slight deviation in that the first, second, and third larval stages develop and remain in the egg until a set of yet-to-be-determined extra-egg conditions (temperature changes and physical abrasion are implicated) induce hatching of the infective L3. Egg confinement of the larvae seems to enable pasture forms to persist for extensive periods in the northern tier of the United States [22]. *Nematodirus* is a dose-limiting nematode for macrocyclic lactones, but because of the rapid development of immunologic resistance to this pathogenic worm, problematic populations developed in the wake of macrocyclic lactone usage do not appear to be of significant dimension in commercial cattle operations as opposed to the situation with the cooperiads.

Strongyloides papillosus is parasitic in the small intestine as a population of parthenogenetic females, resulting in infections during heterogonic and homogonic life cycles. Cattle become infected by transmammary, transcutaneous, and oral routes of larval acquisition. This species is eclipsed in the literature by its fellow species of *S westeri*, *S ransomi*, and *S stercoralis*, which infect horses, swine, and dogs (plus humans), respectively. The eggs of *S papillosus* are small and light colored relative to strongyle eggs, and are seemingly of increased numbers in fecal flotations immediately after anthelmintic treatment. In reality, treatment results in the removal of the strongyle eggs thereby rendering the *Strongyloides* eggs more noticeable (Yazwinski, personal observation). *Strongyloides* burdens are rarely of a pathogenic nature in cattle, with transmission of greatest proportion during wet conditions that facilitate the transcutaneous route of infection (confined or feedlot cattle) [23].

Oesophagostomum radiatum is the nodular worm of cattle and can infect transcutaneously (tracheal migration) and *per os*. Fourth-stage larvae reside in submucosal nodules in the small intestine and adults populate the proximal large intestine. This nematode is of high farm but low individual animal incidence as determined by coproculture. Very low nematode counts per animal are the rule. Although seemingly inductive of extensive host sensitization (systemic migration) and tissue reaction (intestinal nodules), cattle do not become protectively immune, with infections of adult animals being relatively common, albeit light [17].

Pasture-level nematode populations

The stages and their locations

On pasture, GI nematode populations proceed from egg to first, second, and third larval stages. With each defecation a sequential progression starts anew. An appreciation for the dimension of these pasture inoculations with preparasitic stages can be obtained from work done in Minnesota, where several cow–calf pairs were continuously scrutinized from calving to weaning for the quantification of defecation patterns during the 205-day suckling period [24]. It was determined that an adult cow produces 4.4 times more feces that does its weanling calf (16.2 kg versus 3.7 kg of feces per day). In accordance with the above fecal production and coincident nematode egg counts, it was further established that cows deposited 33% more eggs onto the pasture than did their calves, and that each cow–calf pair accounted for 5×10^6 eggs added to the pasture per suckling period. Given the size of the cow–calf industry in the United States (approximately 30 million mature cows) [25], the fact that the cow–calf industry is only a section of beef production in the United States (dairy production is likewise strapped by nematode parasites), and the tendency that nematode parasitisms increase in magnitude as one progresses from Minnesota to the south and southeast United States where the cow–calf industry is centered, one can only imagine the enormity of parasite reservoirs that are continuously supplemented on pastures each grazing season.

Obviously, not all deposited eggs are ultimately realized as cattle parasites. In fact, most eggs do not result in infective larvae on herbage. In a lengthy set of studies in Louisiana, approximately 3% of voided eggs were ultimately available as infective larvae on pasture herbage [26,27]. Attrition was most acute during the development from egg to L2. The above researchers and others noted that the normal extent of lateral migration is 15 cm from the original site of pat disposition [28], with some migration as far as 30 cm. These measures of larval contamination relative to the site of dung deposition were from undisturbed feces. Various means of physical dispersal (eg, splashing rain, coprophagous beetle activity, wind, animal traffic, pasture dragging, bird foraging) would expand the zone of contamination and animal exposure.

Just as lateral larval migration from the point of initial egg deposition is influenced by several factors [29], vertical migration likewise is subject to several determinants (eg, herbage type, nematode species, surface moisture, temperature). Vertical migration in Louisiana was noted to extend as high as 8 cm [26], a migration that was enabled by warm, moist conditions.

Determinants of pasture-stage success

Several excellent discussions on the factors that influence nematode development and survival on pasture have been written and should be accessed if additional information in this area is needed [24,30,31]. The major determinants for pasture stage success are discussed below.

Temperature and moisture

These are the most influential and critical determinants. Optimum and essential ranges of both determinants have been demonstrated for stage development, survival, migration, and infectivity. Duration of species-specific intolerable temperatures (cold or hot) determines a nematode's range in the United States. Generally, temperatures required for nematode development and survival are between 6° and 35°C [32], with an optimal temperature range of 7° to 25°C if survivability is considered also [26,27].

Adequate moisture is as important as critical temperature for nematode success on pasture. In multiple-year studies, researchers documented the absolute necessity of moisture (fecal and atmospheric) for larval development and translation onto surrounding herbage [33,34]. In Louisiana, initial fecal water content was correlated with the rate at which L3 were freed from the feces soon after deposition [27]. Release of reservoir larvae from older dung pats was noted to occur in relation to rain, primarily in the form of thunderstorms [26].

Miscellaneous ambient conditions

Sunlight and shade, air flow, transpiration, snow cover, herbage type, microenvironment of the pasture mat, and soil type relative to moisture-holding ability all influence the success of pasture-level nematode populations.

Pasture flora and fauna

The pasture mat and dung should be viewed as a teeming brew of living forms superimposed onto the cow–herbage working system—a collection of organisms that ultimately facilitate the pasture ecosystem. Included are: bacteria and protozoa, which aid in the degradation of feces and nutrient supply to developing nematodes; a multitude of fungi, both commensal and predaceous toward nematode life stages; coprophilic diptera, coleoptera, and micro-arthropods (Mesostigmata) that feed off and within pasture mat and dung; annelids, which are capable of processing upward of 95% of a pasture's dung within 50 days of deposition and thereby greatly reducing the levels of L3 on herbage; and larger life forms, such as birds (eg, cowbirds, egrets) [35–37].

Of the natural cohabitants of pasture and pasture dung listed above, two have been cited for their extensive influence on nematode life stage survival and success: predaceous fungi and coprophagous beetles [37]. Approximately 200 species of fungi have been shown to be predaceous on pasture nematodes, with lethal action in the forms of ovicide, endoparasitism, and trapping. The fungal species *Duddingtonia flagrans* has received the greatest attention in efforts to effect biologic control of nematode challenge, with upward of 80% reduction of pasture L3 in some studies [38]. Several conditions have to be stringently maintained for fungal control to be successful, conditions that are out of bounds for husbandry or cultural manipulation, such as fecal moisture and temperature. Generally, conditions that optimize nematode success negatively affect fungal growth and activity [31].

Coprophagous beetles are collectively a major component in the potential management of cattle dung, pasture fertility, and nematode life stages [39]. These industrious arthropods invade and use dung in various patterns characterized as tumbling, tunneling, and dwelling, at all times consuming and moving feces, thereby removing nematode life stages from the cycle of infectivity and eventual parasitism. Given the natural and beneficial presence of coprophagous beetles on cattle pastures, it is not surprising that the adverse effects of certain endectocides have been cited. It seems that the avermectin-series macrocyclic lactones are markedly detrimental to coprophilic beetles, with eprinomectin being the most offensive [40,41]. Controlled and spatially or temporally circumspect studies detail marked detriment of avermectins on beetle activity (reproduction and development), but similarly alarming observations made in the natural setting (ie, moderating effects of reservoir beetles) have not been forthcoming.

Pasture-stage longevity

Persistence of free-living stages on pasture is extremely varied and directly dependent on nematode species, moisture, temperature, and protection from the direct and indirect lethal actions of fungi, protozoa, mites, beetles, other nematodes, birds, and mammals. Studies document L3 survival on pasture as ranging from mere days to years [42,43]. Extensive work in Louisiana documented larval longevity in the southeastern quadrant of the United States [26,27]. Infective L3 persisted for the greatest period (8 months) when conditions were cool and wet (October to May) but died off within weeks during the summer after rain-induced liberation from dung pats. Infective larvae acquired by grazing cattle during the summer months were from recently deposited feces, and no significant reservoiring of life stages occurs in the summer because of the extremely high temperatures and only sporadic rainfall.

In the northern tier of the United States, neither dryness nor high temperatures are encountered routinely by nematode life stages for extensive periods as is common in the south. As a result, nematode longevity in the north is longer, with recovery of L3 from herbage extending for 12 months after egg deposition for most trichostrongyle genera [44]. Overwintering of L3 on pasture is the norm in the north, except for *H placei*, which seems to overwinter in an arrested carrier state in infected cattle.

In a 2-year study conducted in Maine [22], pastures were naturally contaminated in the summer and grazed by tracer calves for 2-week intervals starting at 12 and 24 months postcontamination (Fig. 1). Significant levels of challenge were seen at 12 months postcontamination for *Nematodirus* and *Cooperia*, with *Nematodirus* still persisting on pasture after 24 months. *Ostertagia* contamination was evident at low levels for up to 14 months postcontamination. These lengthy durations of larval persistence in the north clearly demonstrate the remote feasibility of providing safe pasture by simply allowing pastures to remain idle. Combined with pasture rest, the following have been suggested as means by which pastures might be decontaminated to the point of being termed safe [26,45]:

Alternating land use as pasture and crop for 2- to 3-year periods
Annual or biannual pasture renovation
Pasture depopulation during months of highest transmission
Cograzing with alternate, less suitable hosts
Avoidance of over-stocking
Supplemental feeding

Prevalence and degrees of GI nematodosis

Overriding determinants

As was the case with the success of environmental stages, many factors collectively dictate the extent to which animals acquire and subsequently

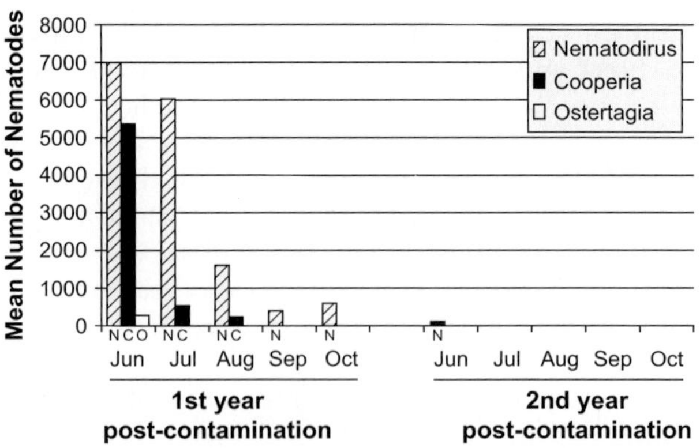

Fig. 1. Mean numbers of nematodes recovered from tracer calves grazed for 2 weeks on plots contaminated 1 to 2 years earlier. (*Data from* Gibbs, HC. Persistence on pasture of infective larvae of nematodes parasitizing Maine dairy cattle. Am J Vet Res 1980;51:1694–5.)

retain nematode parasites (Box 1). Overriding factors serve to determine which nematode species are indigenous to an area and successful in the long term. Animal-, pasture-, and treatment-oriented factors influence and contribute to the extent species-specific infections occur.

In the broad sense, climate determines the prevalence of the parasites, whereas weather dictates the timing of the corresponding parasitisms [46]. The United States experiences a temperate climate and as such supports the parasitisms that can cycle within those ambient conditions. Yearly

Box 1. Determinants of the prevalence and degree of cattle nematodosis

Nature of challenge

Overriding determinants
- Climate
- Weather
- Season
- Region

Pasture and management determinants
- Pasture quality and productivity
- Pasture type
- Pasture topography and drainage
- Grazing management: age group separation, alternate species, stocking rates, rotation, supplemental feeding
- Production type: dairy (confined versus pastured), beef (stocker versus cow/calf versus feedlot, etc)

Animal-based determinants
- Immunologic status
- Physiologic status
- Health

Nature of parasiticidal effort

Effectiveness of parasiticide usage
- Effectiveness of product: spectrum of activity, larvicidal versus adulticidal, degree of resistance
- Persistence of product
- Diminished efficacy: formulation considerations (topicals versus injectables, etc), dietary considerations (gut flow, ingredients, closures, etc), generics

Coordination of epidemiology with treatment

Time and extent of posttreatment challenge

weather patterns relative to temperature and moisture vary on a regional basis across the United States and as a result effect different patterns of parasite prevalence and abundance [47]. *Cooperia* spp and *O ostertagi* predominate across the entire United States. *Trichostrongylus axei, O radiatum*, and *N helvetianus* also blanket the United States but at levels usually much reduced from those established by *Cooperia* or *Ostertagia*. *Haemonchus* spp flourish in the southern plains, limited by the susceptibility of their free-living stages to low environmental temperatures. Sweeping statements characterizing the incidence and epidemiology of cattle nematodes are possible for the northern region, the southern plains region, and the southeastern region. The western quadrant of the United States, however, cannot be ascribed any succinct characterization because of the extremely diverse environmental conditions relative to free-living stage development, longevity, and success (eg, arid versus extremely wet, irrigated versus natural, valley versus mountain, coastal versus inland, and extremely hot versus extremely cold). In regard to parasite intensity, it is generally considered that GI nematode parasitisms are most profound in the southeastern United States because of year-round grazing, ambient conditions of temperature and moisture that permit relatively uninterrupted transmission, vigorous cow–calf and stocker industries, and the presence of all nematode species indigenous to the United States [14,48]. In contrast, cattle raised in northern and western regions generally experience less intensive parasitisms because of lengthy periods of diminished or extinguished transmission (winter snow cover and cold), low stocking rates and cattle populations, and a less extensive incidence of parasite species.

The prevalence of parasitisms in the United States is profound. In a study in Georgia [49], the incidence of *Ostertagia*, *T axei*, *Haemonchus*, and *Cooperia* in 145 cattle were 100%, 97%, 66%, and 63%, respectively. In a 2-year study in Maine [50], only 1 of 263 animals was shown not to display nematode patencies as detected by coprological examinations. Strongyle-type eggs were the most commonly encountered, followed in decreasing order of incidence by *Strongyloides*, *Bunostomum*, *Nematodirus*, *Trichuris*, and *Capillaria* (Fig. 2), an egg-count profile that is for the most part (exception being *Bunostomum*) consistent with that seen across the United States. By way of coproculture, the strongyle eggs voided by the younger animals over this same timeframe were indirectly identified and quantified to strongyle genus (Fig. 3). Except for *Haemonchus* spp calculated EPG counts, which would certainly be of greater magnitude in the south, the relative proportions are generally similar to those that would be displayed across the United States: *Cooperia* spp and *O ostertagi* being predominant, followed in order by *Haemonchus*, *Trichostrongylus*, and *Oesophagostomum*. Seasonality of egg count levels is also evident for each of the strongyle genera (see Fig. 3).

Fundamental epidemiologic patterns also occur with respect to age (Fig. 4). Animals of all age groups started the grazing season with reduced egg counts reflective of a preceding period of low transmission in the winter.

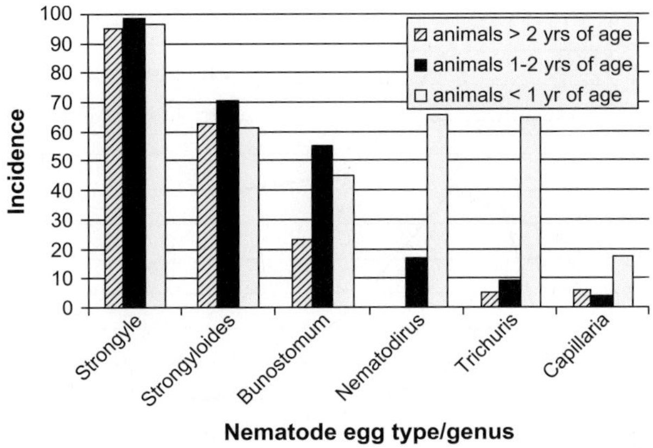

Fig. 2. Mean incidence of patencies, as demonstrated by fecal egg flotation (10-g samples) for dairy animals of different age groups on day 0 and sampled bimonthly over a year's period of time in Maine. (*Data from* Yazwinski TA, Gibbs HC. Survey of helminth infections in Maine dairy cattle. Am J Vet Res 1975;36:1677–82.)

Subsequently, EPG counts were elevated during the grazing season because of contamination, adequate moisture, and temperature. At the end of the grazing season, EPG levels decreased because of reduced temperature for transmission and the fact that the animals were becoming increasingly resistant. This epidemiologic pattern was even more evident in younger animals raised on farms where few, if any, parasite control measures were used (Fig. 5) and the parasitisms could assume the levels as dictated by the natural determinants (eg, climate, season, animal age). On farms where parasite control was a conscious management objective, parasitisms were kept at low levels, as determined by egg counts, for the entire grazing season.

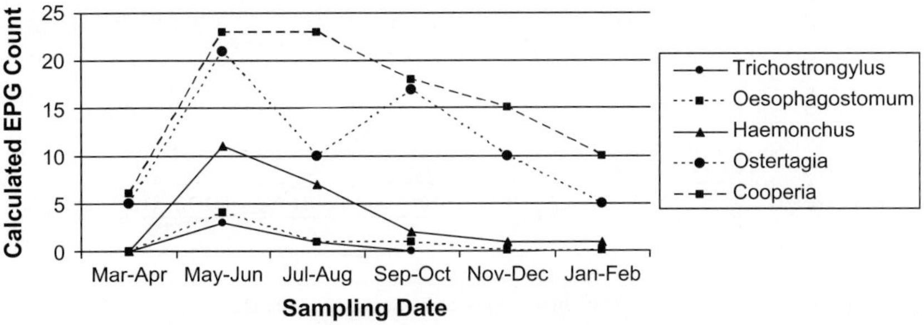

Fig. 3. Genus-specific EPG counts as calculated from strongyle EPG counts and coproculture harvests for Maine dairy replacement cattle 2 years of age or younger at the start of the survey. (*Data from* Yazwinski TA, Gibbs HC. Survey of helminth infections in Maine dairy cattle. Am J Vet Res 1975;36:1677–82.)

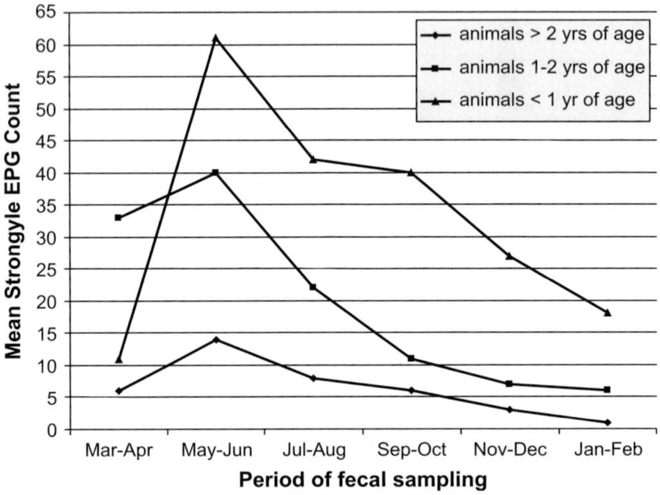

Fig. 4. Mean Strongyle EPG counts by dairy animal age group (at start) and sample date in Maine. (*Data from* Yazwinski TA, Gibbs HC. Survey of helminth infections in Maine dairy cattle. Am J Vet Res 1975;36:1677–82.)

In the previous discussion, the epidemiology of cattle parasitisms was deduced from fecal egg counts and coprocultures. In subsequent work from the same region wherein tracer calves were used [51], it was shown further that low pasture contamination in the spring resulted in subsequent patencies that provided a supply of pasture-level forms for the summer and elevated transmission in the fall, a season-to-season epidemiologic scenario that is typical for many parts of the United States [42]. *Haemonchus* spp infections in the north are the exception, with the lack of overwintering

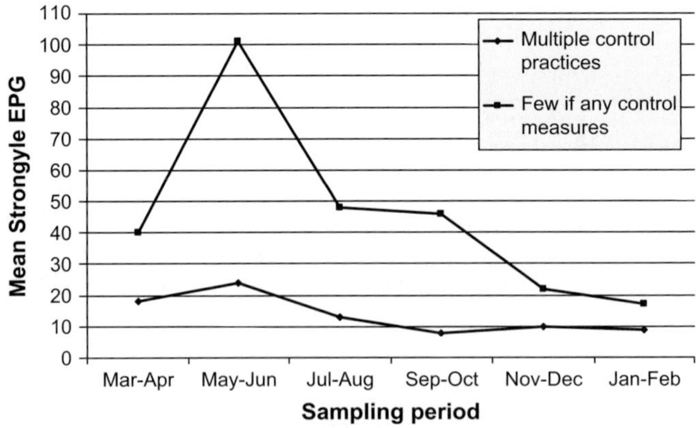

Fig. 5. Strongyle EPG counts for replacement dairy cattle (≤2 years of age in March/April) by sampling period and overall degree of parasite control practices. (*Data from* Yazwinski TA, Gibbs HC. Survey of helminth infections in Maine dairy cattle. Am J Vet Res 1975;36:1677–82.)

pasture stages necessitating long generation time (prepatent plus patent) or newly introduced, infected animals to carry infections from one grazing season to the next.

A tracer calf study conducted on permanent pastures in California yielded results similar to the ones reported from Maine [18]. Low levels of challenge were present in the beginning of the grazing season (December–February) for *Cooperia* and *Ostertagia* (Fig. 6). Immediately thereafter (March–April), elevated levels of challenge were evident. Subsequently, transmission was reduced greatly during the summer followed by a second peak period of transmission and infection in the fall. *Haemonchus* transmission in California was also similar to that seen in Maine, with no challenge in the spring followed by extensive summer and fall pasture contamination and infectivity.

In addition to identifying transmission patterns in California for *Ostertagia*, *Cooperia*, and *Haemonchus*, patterns of arrestment were also demonstrated for these three genera. True seasonal arrestments were apparent for *Ostertagia* and *Haemonchus*, with *Ostertagia* inhibiting in the late spring and early summer and inhibition of ingested *Haemonchus* larvae occurring in the autumn. For *Cooperia*, no seasonal pattern was detected; rather there was a tendency for inhibition to be aligned with intensity of infection [18,52].

As noted previously, *O ostertagi* is the nematode species of most dramatic and structured seasonal arrestment. The dynamics of *Ostertagia* inhibition have been most extensively studied in Louisiana. In a 3-year, two-site study with bimonthly necropsies of sentinel cattle, the consistent patterns of seasonal *Ostertagia* inhibition were documented with peak seasonal arrestment from spring to early summer (Fig. 7) [53]. Interestingly, the high numbers of IEL_4 never evolved into equally as impressive numbers of DL_4 and adults after inhibition was dismissed. Resumed development was mostly of a gradual nature with extensive loss of forms between the IEL_4 and DL_4 stages and the relative lack of classic type II ostertagiasis. Others have also noted that type II ostertagiasis is not a common phenomenon in the United States whether maturation is after summer or winter inhibition [51,54].

Pasture and management determinants

Numerous pasture and animal management factors determine the extent of nematode challenge on farms. The more facilitated the life cycle of the parasite, the greater the dimensions assumed by the nematode parasite at each stage of its life cycle. Pasture quality and productivity are inversely related to parasitisms, all other factors remaining constant. Unfortunately, because of economics and negative effects of pasture overgrowth relative to herbage quality and productivity, the tendency is for high-quality and high-producing pastures also to have high stocking rates. The higher the stocking rates, the greater the propensity for parasite acquisition. Pasture type, topography, and drainage also directly influence the success and

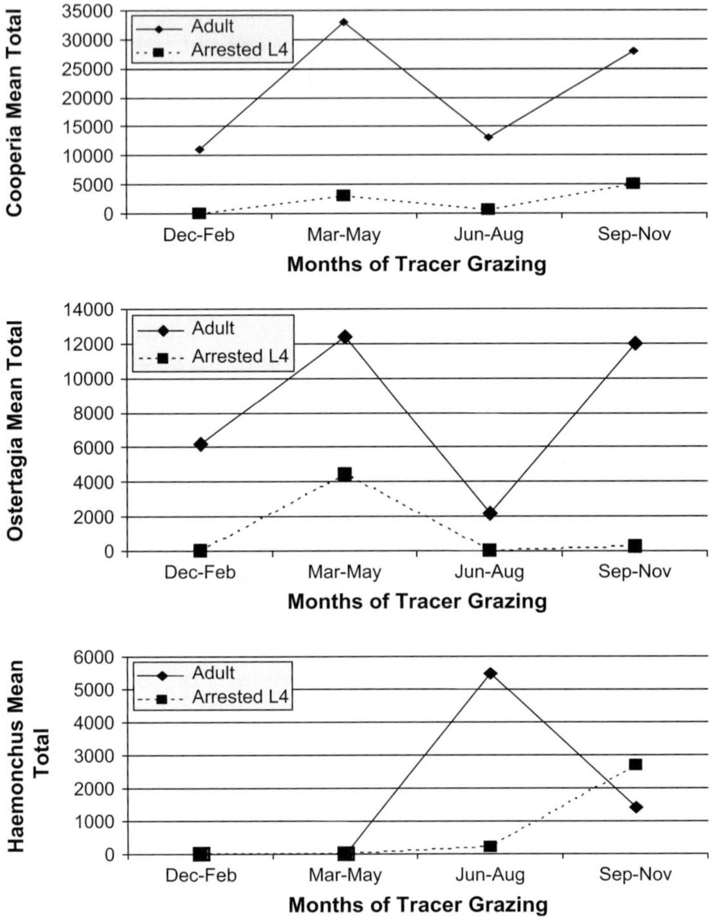

Fig. 6. Levels of nematode adults and arrested fourth-stage larvae in tracer calves placed on irrigated pasture in California. (*Data from* Baker HF, Fisk RA, Bushnell RB, et al. Seasonal occurrence of infective nematode larvae on irrigated pasture grazed by cattle in California. Am J Vet Res 1981;42:1188–91.)

infective potential of the nematode stages on the pasture by determining the pasture mat microclimate relative to moisture and the ease by which L3 might ascend herbage to a level being grazed by the cattle.

Various forms of grazing management have been cited as contributing to rates of nematode acquisition and as such have been recommended as means by which sustainable parasite control might be augmented [26]. Examples include: (1) age group grazing assignments wherein safe pastures are designated for the young animals and older animals are used to clean pastures, (2) stocking rate manipulation, (3) pasture rotation or strip grazing, (4) supplemental feeding, and (5) grazing alternate species. Use of the above, in part or in total, requires a farm-level appreciation for GI parasitisms, the management skills

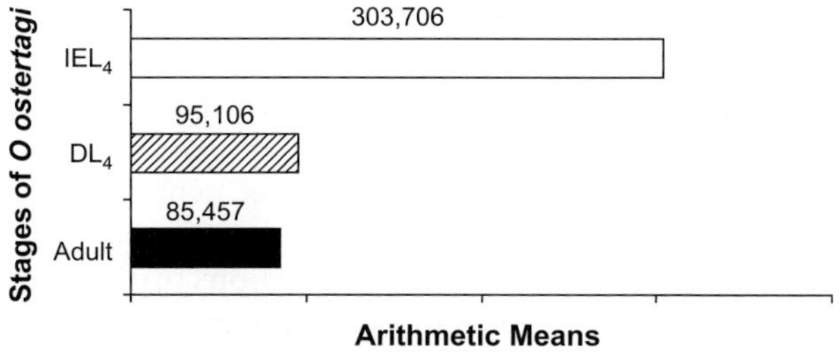

Fig. 7. Peak arithmetic means of sequentially-evolved stages of *O ostertagi* as noted at bimonthly necropsies of sentinel cattle at two locations in Louisiana from 1978–1980. (*Data from* William JC, Knox JW, Baumann BA, et al. Seasonal changes of gastrointestinal nematode populations in yearling beef cattle in Louisiana with emphasis on prevalence of inhibition in *Ostertagia ostertagi.* Int J Parasit 1983;13:133–43.)

and personnel to effect cultural manipulations, and the facilities to accomplish the tasks. In the United States, managerial schemes for parasite control usually are not applied, in favor of doing nothing at all or applying chemical control with extremely varied levels of strategy and effectiveness.

Grazing cattle with alternate, dead-end hosts has been evaluated as a means of parasite control. In several studies, the bovine burdens of *Cooperia* and *Ostertagia* were greatly reduced by cograzing with sheep, but predictably, the levels of *Haemonchus* and *T colubriformis* were elevated [55,56]. In another study lasting over 3 years, cograzing calves with older cattle proved a much greater deterrent to parasite acquisition than grazing calves with sheep (Fig. 8) [57]. Additionally, the levels of sentinel calf parasitisms were manipulated to a greater extent by rainfall as opposed to either method of grazing control. In the United States, cograzing alternate species is

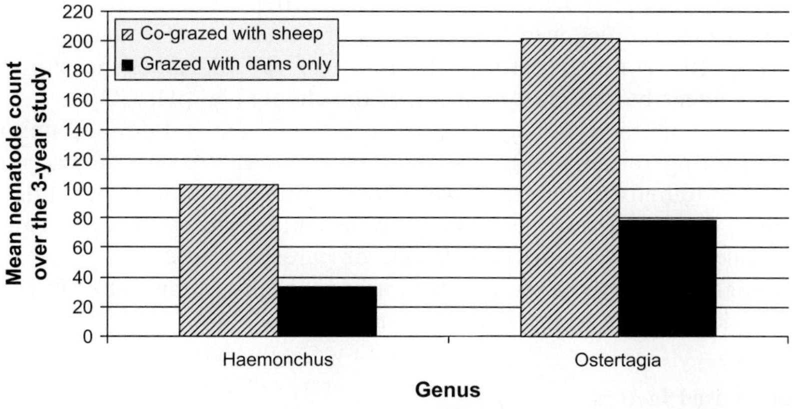

Fig. 8. Mean levels of nematodes in calves grazed from spring to fall with their dams alone or in combination with ewe–lamb pairs (9 calves/yr for years 1983, 1984, and 1985). (*Data from* Jordan HE, Phillips WA, Morrison RD, et al. A 3-year study of continuous mixed grazing of cattle and sheep: parasitism of offspring. Int J Parasit 1988;18:779–4.)

common on small farms where beef or dairy production is not intensely practiced. For commercial operations, cograzing is not seen as a feasible measure for parasite control because of managerial and facility incompatibility coupled with producer prejudice.

Perhaps one of the greatest pasture and management determinants of parasite prevalence is that of production type: dairy versus beef. Within each of these production types, additional inherent variations further modify and dictate levels of animal parasitism. On dairies, the extent of pasture usage and resultant parasite burdens vary on a farm and animal-age basis. Animal grazing schemes range from zero grazing to full time, with degree of parasitism directly correlated with degree of pasture usage [23]. Beef animals, regardless of age, are continuously on pasture before their eventual placement at feedlots for finishing. Parasite burdens are gained early in the animal's life and maintained throughout the entire grazing phase because of continuous challenge and a general lack of complete immunologic protection [58]. Some infections are acquired early that do render the animals immunologically refractory to future infections (*Nematodirus* and *Dictyocaulus*). *Cooperia* spp infections are common and of significant magnitude for the first two complete grazing seasons only, with low-level infections common for the remainder of the animal's life [59]. The abomasal genera (*Ostertagia*, *Trichostrongylus*, and *Haemonchus*) persist in abundance regardless of age group.

Parasite burdens are acquired by beef calves during the nursing phase, with the dam's mothering ability (milk provision) inversely related to the size and activity of nursing calf parasite burdens. In a 2-year study comparing parasitisms of calves under ad libitum and restricted nursing regions (Fig. 9), the restriction of suckling significantly increased parasite burdens by *Ostertagia*, *T axei*, and *Cooperia* as measured by EPG counts [60]. In another study, calves fed milk only versus those fed milk and roughage were given standardized inoculates of *O ostertagi* [61]. Both worm acquisition and worm fecundities were enhanced by the addition of roughage to the diet (Fig. 10), considered to be the result of reticulorumen development and coincident biochemical qualities of the chyme (eg, pH, CO_2).

Parasite burdens generally decrease as animals age and develop immune competence against challenge infections. In addition, it is generally accepted that dairy animals experience lower parasite burdens than do beef animals because of grazing restriction and supplemental feeding characteristic of dairy animal management [51]. Levels of parasite burdens in adult dairy cows might therefore be viewed as indicative of the lower end of infection magnitudes that naturally occur in cattle (Table 2) [17].

Animal-based factors

Animal health, immunologic status and physiologic state influence parasite acquisition, retention, and activity. Immunologic response to GI parasites is primarily humoral, and all factors that negatively affect the Th2 response

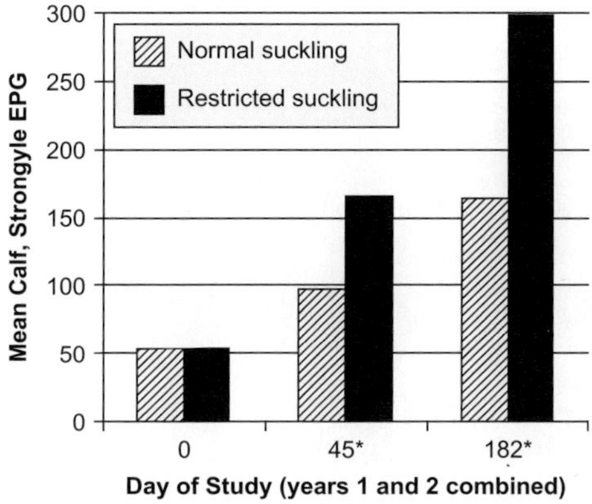

Fig. 9. Strongyle EPG counts for beef calves under normal or restricted suckling schemes. (*indicates egg counts significantly different [$P = 0.05$]). (*Data from* Ciordia H, Stuedemann JA, Wilkinson SR, et al. Effect of a once-daily suckling program on gastrointestinal parasitism in Angus cows and calves. Am J Vet Res 1985;46:566–9.)

mechanism in turn compromise the immune regulation of nematode parasitisms. Integral to the immune response are IgG1 [62], IgE [63], activated complement, and specifically mobilized eosinophils [64]. In addition, nonspecific inflammatory and hyperplastic responses at the site of tissue invasion and irritation by the parasite serve to limit parasite development.

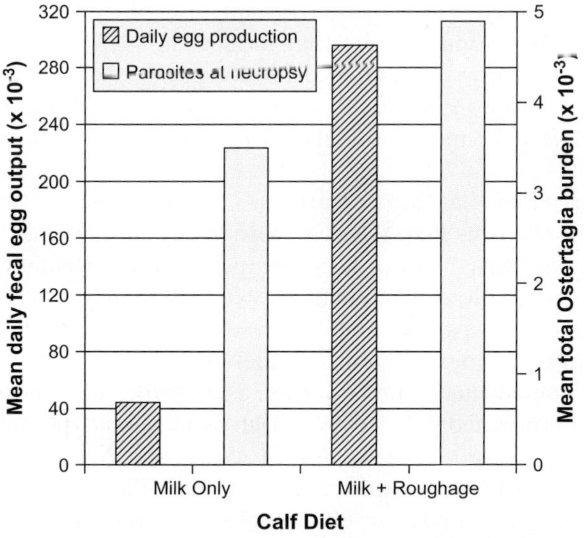

Fig. 10. Levels of egg output and established *Ostertagia* following identical larval administration to calves of divergent diet and reticulorumen development. (*Data from* Satrigia F, Nanson P, Christensen CM. *Ostertagia ostertagi* in neonatal calves: establishment of infection in ruminating and non-ruminating calves. Res Vet Sci 1991;51:344–6.)

Table 2
Nematodes recovered at the necropsy of 10 untreated dairy cows during May of 1998 in Arkansas

Site	Nematode	Prevalence	Range	Geometric mean
Abomasum	*O ostertagi*			
	adult	10/10	353–14570	2167
	IEL_4	10/10	321–77614	8648
	T axei	10/10	114–16775	743
	H placei	2/10	0–17	1
Small intestine	*Cooperia*			
	spp ♀	9/10	0–5956	105
	punctata ♂	6/10	0–3894	9
	oncophora ♂	5/10	0–1380	18
	surnabada ♂	3/10	0–127	3
Large intestine	*O radiatum*	5/10	0–26	1
	Trichuris sp	1/10	0–2	1

Data from Yazwinski TA, Tucker C, Copeland S, et al. Dose confirmation of moxidectin pour-on against natural nematode infections in lactating dairy cattle. Vet Parasitol 1999; 86:223–8.

Female cattle display a greater degree of immune regulation of GI parasitisms than do males, evidently the result of a more constructive nature of estrogens as opposed to androgens in regard to immune system development [65]. This gender-oriented immune competence is most demonstrable in adults and is temporarily lessened at parturition and the beginning of lactation as part of the periparturient rise phenomenon [22,66]. All physiologic or hormonal factors that induce this depressed immune state have not been identified, but corticosteroids and prolactin appear to be involved in a hyporesponsiveness in the host with lowered populations of effector T and B cells and ultimately lowered specific antibody production [65,67].

It is often stated that 20% of a farm's animal population cycles 60%–80% of the parasitisms [68]. Fecal nematode egg counts and post-necropsy parasite enumerations from cattle of common rearing repeatedly display this non-normal distribution of parasitisms within host populations. Additionally, immunologic resistance to GI nematodes is a heritable characteristic with a heritability index of approximately 0.30. In a study conducted in Maryland, calves of high and low EPG phenotypes were necropsied after cograzing contaminated pasture [62]. High EPG phenotype calves harbored 50% more *O ostertagi*, *C oncophora*, *H placei*, and *N helvetianus* than did their low EPG phenotype counterparts (Fig. 11). Parasite levels were negatively correlated with IgG1, an effector element that was mostly under the influence of sires.

Although genetically conferred immunologic reactivity is a proven occurrence and of measurable benefit in small ruminant production, the use of genetic selection for parasite control in cattle populations is not envisioned as

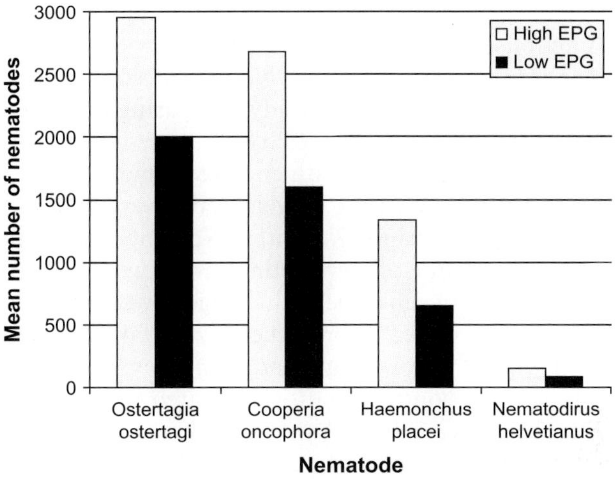

Fig. 11. Mean numbers of naturally acquired nematodes in weaned calves of either high or low EPG phenotypes and sire groups. (*Data from* Gasbarre LC, Leighton EA, Davies CJ. Genetic control of immunity to gastrointestinal nematodes of cattle. Vet Parasit 1990;37:257–72.)

probable [69]. Reasons given for this pessimistic outlook include the long generation time with cattle, low cattle reproduction rates (dam side), difficulty in timely assessment of resistant phenotypes (and genotypes), and the probability that parasites will readily adapt to effective immune responses through selection and reproduction. In addition, the degree of control that might be possible through genetic selection of the host may not restrict the level of worm detriment to a point that it is acceptable to the producer.

Parasiticidal efforts and effects

Temporary reprieve from GI nematode infections is accomplished, to varying degrees, by chemical intervention with one of the multitude of products that are available today (>40) for commercial use in cattle. Although the choices are bountiful, only a few drug classes are represented in the United States: imidazothiazole (levamisole), benzimidazole (oxfendazole, albendazole, and fenbendazole), and macrocyclic lactone (ivermectin, doramectin, eprinomectin, and moxidectin). All of the above compounds vary from one another in spectrum of activity, therapeutic efficacy, and remnant (persistent) efficacy. Additionally, they confer varying degrees of stage-specific efficacy (adulticidal versus larvicidal, developing versus inhibited).

Results from nematocide usage pertaining to efficacy and enhanced animal performance are extremely varied, and published reports can be found that document the effectiveness of each compound as equal to or better than any other compound. Two of the most popular compounds in the United

States are fenbendazole and ivermectin, a situation that has been evident for many years (unpublished survey data, Arkansas Extension Service, 2000). Because of their prominence, these two parasiticides have been the targets of many market support studies. One study comparing the two for effectiveness also yielded data indicating the ability of these products to alter parasite transmission (Fig. 12) [70]. Treatment group mean EPG counts were consistent; ivermectin every 6 weeks < ivermectin every 12 weeks < fenbendazole < control when grazed for 7 months (November through May). The suppressive treatment regime of ivermectin every 6 weeks clearly prevented pasture contamination and subsequent challenge. Twelve-week intervals between treatments with ivermectin or fenbendazole failed to reduce pasture contamination. Despite a preceding 6 months of extensive contamination from resident calves, the control pastures appeared to lose challenge intensity as measured by tracer calves. Assuredly, the control pastures did not lose infective stage contamination to a greater extent than did the other pastures, but rather the tracer calf method of contamination assessment was shown to be faulty in this instance. The control pasture tracer burdens also further illustrated the varied and unpredictable nature of parasite acquisition and retention.

An Arkansas study compared fenbendazole (10 and 5 mg/kg bodyweight (BW) on days 0 and 56, respectively, or 10 mg/kg BW on day 0 only) to injectable ivermectin for the control of stocker calf parasitism [71]. The higher dosage of fenbendazole was used on day 0 because of the assumed elevated burdens of *Ostertagia* IEL_4 in Arkansas in July [53]. Control (no treatment)

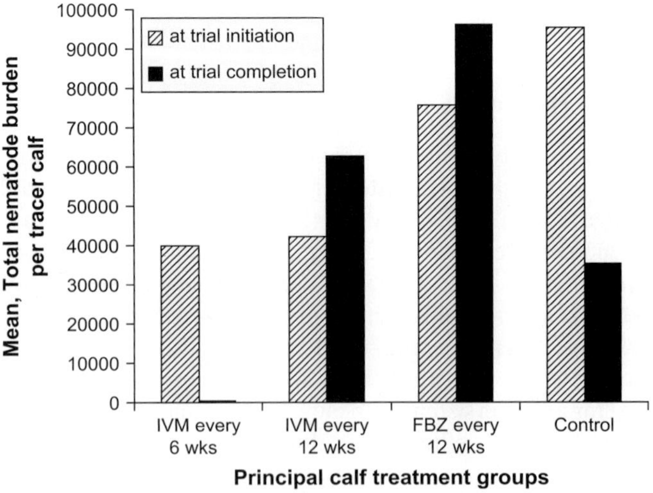

Fig. 12. Mean total tracer calf nematode burdens after grazing principal pastures for 18 days at trial initiation (November, 1986) and completion (May, 1987) in Louisiana. (*Data from* Williams JC, Knox JW, Barras SA, et al. Effects of ivermectin and fenbendazole in strategic treatment of GI nematode infections in cattle. Am J Vet Res 1990;51:2034–43.)

and ivermectin sustained release bolus (ISRB) treatment groups also were included to illustrate the degrees of parasitism that develop in stockers if there is no chemical intervention or if there is complete suppressive therapy. For the entire 133-day study, the ISRB-treated calves shed no or few strongyle eggs (Fig. 13). Conversely, control animals exhibited the highest EPG counts for the entire study. Egg count levels for the fenbendazole and ivermectin treatment groups were depressed immediately after treatment, but rebounded soon thereafter. All fenbendazole treatments resulted in significant egg count reductions as noted at 28 days posttreatment ($P < 0.05$), whereas only the day 0 ivermectin treatments were followed by significant EPG count reductions. Given the extreme difference in egg shedding by control and ISRB calves during the 133-day study, tracer calves were placed on their pastures the following spring to determine the degree to which residual challenge may be dictated by extent of prior year parasite control (Fig. 14). Tracer calves that grazed ISRB pastures acquired burdens of *O ostertagi* (adults and IEL_4), *Cooperia* spp, and *T axei* that were greatly reduced from those harbored by calves that grazed the control pasture, clearly underscoring the merits of parasite control in regard to residual challenge encountered by the next year's naïve animals.

The above studies depicted various degrees of nematode control that may be induced by some of the products available today. Nematocide usage is routinely met with varying degrees of success because of several contributing factors [72]. Decreased drug efficacy may result from: (1) use of a product at epidemiologically inappropriate times, (2) administration of a product at incorrect dosages, (3) nematode resistance, and (4) animal-level modifications of effective drug levels, including rate of gut passage, rumen microbe biotransformations, gut-level inflammation, blood protein binding capacity

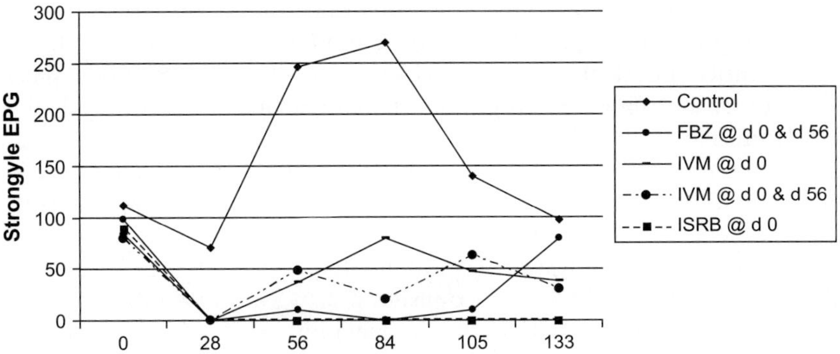

Fig. 13. Strongyle EPG arithmetic means for stocker cattle placed on contaminated pastures from July to November, 1998, in Arkansas. (*Data from* Fincher M, Hubbell D, Tucker C, et al. Current and subsequent season effects of parasite control in Arkansas stocker calves. In: Johnson ZB, Kellogg DW, editors. Arkansas Animal Science Department Report. AR Agri Exp Station Research Series 478; 2000. p. 7–9.)

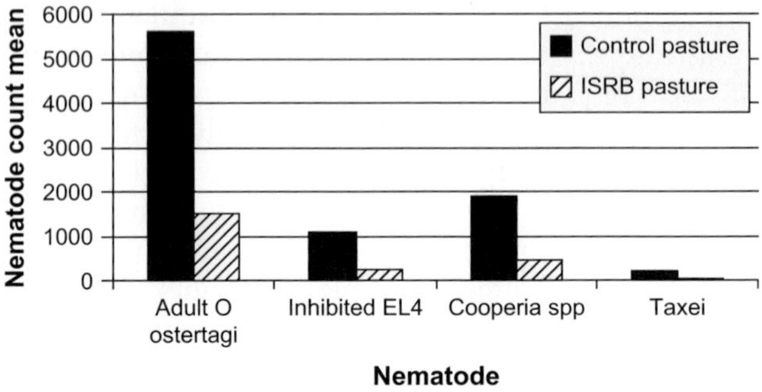

Fig. 14. Tracer calf nematode count arithmetic means ($N = 4$) after grazing previous year's principal pastures for 30 days (March, 2000). (*Data from* Fincher M, Hubbell D, Tucker C, et al. Current and subsequent season effects of parasite control in Arkansas stocker calves. In: Johnson ZB, Kellogg DW, editors. Arkansas Animal Science Department Report. AR Agri Exp Station Research Series 478; 2000. p. 7–9.)

[72], depth of inhibition of *Ostertagia* (for benzimidazoles) [48], self- and allogrooming by animals treated with topicals [73,74], and amount and position of animal fat deposits, which serve to influence availability of the lipophilic macrocyclic lactones [75].

It may be argued that too much reliance is placed on chemical intervention for parasite control in the United States. With the attempted control of any population of gene-based offending organisms, no single means of control is sustainable if survivors are permitted, for at that point it is merely a matter of time for survivor reproduction to reestablish the offending population [76]. With GI nematodes, the existence of survivors after the use of any new nematocide is postulated by some as assured [12], given the tendencies of these nematodes for immense genome quantity and diversity, high mutation rates (especially of mitochondrial DNA, the site of many resistance genes), posttranslational modification of mRNA, the extremely varied physical and physiologic status of each nematode species at any time, and enhanced p-glycoprotein removal of parasiticidal molecules from nematode cells.

With the recent observations of nematode resistance to macrocyclic lactones around the world, including the United States [77], it is apparent that no cattle nematocides are resistance-free [78,79]. Populations resistant to macrocyclic lactones, however, appear limited to species of *Cooperia* and *Haemonchus* [19,80]. Given the extensive use of ivermectin and the other macrocyclic lactones since 1981, it was inevitable that resistance in nematodes would develop to molecules of that compound class [81]. At the time of initial ivermectin availability and for some time thereafter, animal treatment was followed by a 2- to 3-week period of negative fecal egg counts with correspondingly diminished pasture contamination and transmission. Today, treatment with macrocyclic lactones routinely yields fecal egg count reduction (FECR) percentages of 90% or greater, but rarely 100%.

Transmission is reduced but not stopped, and pretreatment levels of egg shedding are soon reestablished. In addition to the extensive use of macrocyclic lactones contributing to resistance, two other factors have been cited: the great popularity of pour-on products, which characteristically and inherently do not allow for appropriate chemical availability [75], and the recent host of competitively-priced generic products, which have extremely varied and, for some, sub-efficacious plasma and tissue concentrations posttreatment [82]. A field study to evaluate various commercial topical ivermectins (including three generic compounds) showed that all pour-ons significantly depressed egg counts, but only two of the four products displayed FECR percentages of 90% or greater [83]. Statistically significant ($P < 0.05$) differences in egg counts (treated versus control group) were evident for 14 days for one generic product, 28 days for the other two generic products, and 42 days for the nongeneric product (Fig. 15). In addition, coproculture revealed that *Haemonchus* eggs were being shed from animals in every generic ivermectin treatment group on day 14, but not from animals treated with the nongeneric compound. It is evident from these data that the generic products were not as effective as the original product, an observation also made by others who suggest a formulation or vehicle basis for the reduced effectiveness [84]. It is curious that generic parasiticides are not evaluated for effectiveness during their abbreviated periods of review by regulatory agencies. If controlled evaluations were required not only would product quality be assured but a timely reassessment of chemical efficacy also would be provided. This is a proverbial Pandora's box suggestion, but controlled evaluation of generics with the original product as a standard would facilitate the detection of resistant strains of parasites at a time when therapies and strategies might be adjusted for resistance curtailment, a much-needed activity for the provision of effective products and correct recommendations.

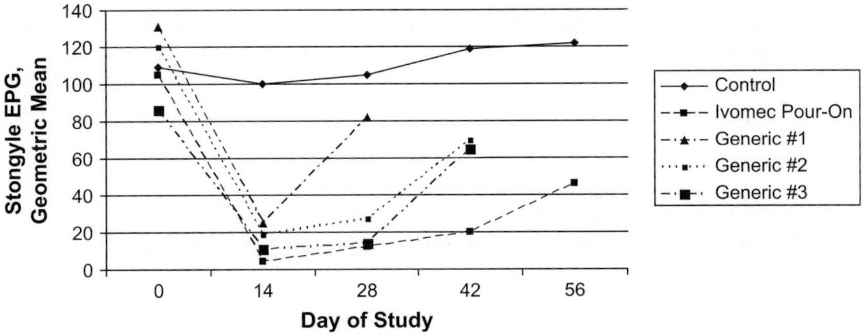

Fig. 15. Strongyle EPG geometric means for control calves and for calves given commercial, topical preparations of ivermectin (Ivomec Pour-On and three generics). (*Data from* Yazwinski TA, Tucker CA, Hornsby JA, et al. A field trial evaluation of several commercial Ivermectin pour-on products in the treatment of cattle nematodiasis. Arkansas Cattle Business 2004; 20(9):44–6.)

Summary

A multitude of factors governs the epidemiology of GI nematodes. In addition, no factor is without influence from others that also manipulate the cycling of parasites. This article is a summary of only a small portion of the research published on nematode epidemiology. Despite all the completed work and all that is know about parasite epidemiology, however, the discipline is still investigative and not predictive. Every sample we read, every trial we run, every statistical analysis we perform, the likelihood of surprise is omnipresent and often fulfilled. We thank the people referenced in this paper, and the many more whose work is equally valuable to this field of science. Their countless hours of work have been productive and vital for the provision of animal health around the world.

References

[1] Levine ND. Nematode parasites of domestic animals and of man. 2nd edition. Minneapolis: Burgess; 1980.
[2] Soulsby EJL. Helminths, arthropods and protozoa of domesticated animals. 7th edition. Philadelphia: Lea & Febiger; 1982.
[3] Marquarat WC, Demaree RS, Grieve RB. Parasitology and vector biology. 2nd edition. San Diego: Academic Press; 2000.
[4] Waller PJ. The future of anthelmintics in sustainable parasite control programs for livestock. Helmithologia 2003;40(2):97–102.
[5] Vercruysse J, Claerebout E. Treatment vs. non-treatment of helminth infections in cattle: defining the threshold. Vet Parasit 2001;98:195–214.
[6] Sangster NC. Managing parasiticide resistance. Vet Parasit 2001;98:89–109.
[7] Shoop WL, Mrozik H, Fisher MH. Structure and activity of avermectins and milbemycins in animal health. Vet Parasitol 1995;59:139–56.
[8] Anderson RC. Nematode parasites of vertebrates: their development and transmission. Wallingford: CAB International; 1992.
[9] Samuel WM, Pybus MJ, Kocan AA. Parasitic diseases of wild mammals. 2nd edition. Ames: Iowa State University Press; 2001.
[10] Bowman DD, Lynn RC, Eberhard ML. Georgi's parasitology for veterinarians. 8th edition. St. Louis: Saunders; 2003.
[11] Myers GH. Avermectin resistance in an Ohio beef cattle herd. In: Proceedings of the 50th Annual Meeting of the American Association of Veterinary Parasitologists. Minneapolis, (MN): 2005; Abstract 44.
[12] Prichard RK. Genetic variability following selection of *Haemonchus contortus* with anthelmintics. Trends Parasitol 2001;17(9):445–53.
[13] Klesius PH. Immunity to *Ostertagia ostertagi*. Vet Parasitol 1988;27:159–67.
[14] Williams JC, Knox JW, Loyacano AF. Epidemiology of *Ostertagia ostertagi* in weaner-yearling cattle. Vet Parasitol 1993;46:313–24.
[15] Frank GR, Herd RP, Marbury KS, et al. Additional investigations on hypobiosis of *Ostertagia ostertagi* after transfer between northern and southern U.S.A. Int J Parasitol 1988;18: 171–7.
[16] Williams JC, Knox JW, Marbury KS, et al. The epidemiology of *Ostertagia ostertagi* and other gastrointestinal nematodes of cattle in Louisiana. Parasitology 1987;95:135–53.
[17] Yazwinski TA, Tucker C, Copeland S, et al. Dose confirmation of moxidectin pour-on against natural nematode infections in lactating dairy cattle. Vet Parasitol 1999;86:223–8.

[18] Baker NF, Fisk RA, Bushnell RB, et al. Seasonal occurrence of infective nematode larvae on irrigated pasture grazed by cattle in California. Am J Vet Res 1981;42:1188–91.
[19] Anziani OS, Suarez V, Guglielmone AA, et al. Resistance to benzimidazole and macrocyclic lactone anthelmintics in cattle nematodes in Argentina. Vet Parasitol 2004;122:303–6.
[20] Anziani OS, Zimmermann G, Guglielmone AA, et al. Avermectin resistance in *Cooperia pectinata* in cattle in Argentina. Vet Rec 2001;149:58–9.
[21] Njue AI, Prichard RK. Efficacy of ivermectin in calves against a resistant *Cooperia oncophora* field isolate. Parasitol Res 2004;93:419–22.
[22] Gibbs HC. Persistence on pasture of infective larvae of nematodes parasitizing Maine dairy cattle. Am J Vet Res 1980;41(10):1694–5.
[23] Herd RP, Riedel RM, Heider LE. Identification and epidemiologic significance of nematodes in a dairy barn. JAVMA 1980;176(12):1370–2.
[24] Stromberg BE. Environmental factors influencing transmission. Vet Parasitol 1997;72: 247–64.
[25] Peel DS. Beef cattle growing and back-grounding programs. Vet Clin Food Animal 2003;19: 365–85.
[26] Williams JC, Bilkovich FR. Distribution of *Ostertagia ostertagi* infective larvae on pasture herbage. Am J Vet Res 1973;34(10):1337–44.
[27] Williams JC, Bilkovich FR. Development and survival of infective larvae of the cattle nematode, *Ostertagia ostertagi.* J Parasitol 1971;57(2):327–38.
[28] Stromberg BE, Averbeck GA. The role of parasite epidemiology in the management of grazing cattle. Int J Parasitol 1999;29:33–9.
[29] Tarshis IB. A preliminary study of the lateral migration by infective larvae of some cattle nematodes on experimentally contaminated forage plots. Proc Helminthol Soc Wash 1958;25(2):99–106.
[30] Waller PJ. Sustainable nematode parasite control strategies for ruminant livestock by grazing management and biological control. Anim Feed Sci Technol 2006;126:277–89.
[31] Waller PJ, Faedo M. The prospects for biological control of the free-living stages of nematode parasites of livestock. Int J Parasitol 1996;26:915–25.
[32] Ciordia H, Bizzell WE. The effects of various constant temperatures on the development of the free-living stages of some nematode parasites of cattle. J Parasitol 1963;49(1):60–3.
[33] Lancaster MB, Hong C. Observations on the pattern of nematode larvae availability on pasture grazed annually by cattle; 1959 to 1985. Vet Rec 1987;120:502–3.
[34] Krecek RC, Murrell KD, Douglass LW. Effects of microclimate variables on the availability and movement of third-stage larvae of *O ostertagi* on herbage. Onder J Vet Res 1990;57: 133–5.
[35] Grønvold J. On the possible role of earthworms in the transmission of *Ostertagia ostertagi* third-stage larvae from feces to soil. J Parasit 1979;65(5):831–2.
[36] Grønvold J. Field experiment on the ability of earthworms (Lumbricidae) to reduce the transmission of infective larvae of *Cooperia oncophora* (Trichostrongylidae) from cow pats to grass. J Parasit 1987;73:1133–7.
[37] Grønvold J, Henriksen SA, Larsen M, et al. Biological control. Aspects of biological control—with special reference to arthropods, protozoans, and helminths of domesticated animals. Vet Parasitol 1996;64:47–64.
[38] Grønvold J, Wolstrup J, Nansen P, et al. Nematode-trapping fungi against parasitic cattle nematodes. Parasitol Today 1993;9(4):137–40.
[39] Fincher GT. Effects of dung beetle activity on the number of nematode parasites acquired by grazing cattle. J Parasitol 1975;61:759–62.
[40] Wardhaugh KG, Longstaff BC, Morton R. A comparison of the development and survival of the dung beetle, *Onthophagus taurus* (Schreb.) when fed on the faeces of cattle treated with pour-on formulations of eprinomectin or moxidectin. Vet Parasitol 2001;99:155–68.
[41] Ridsdill-Smith TJ. Effects of avermectin residues in cattle dung on dung beetle *(Coleoptera: Scarabaeidae)* reproduction and survival. Vet Parasitol 1993;48:127–37.

[42] Michel JF. Observations on the epidemiology of parasitic gastro-enteritis in calves. J Helminthol 1969;43:111–33.
[43] Barger IA, Lewis RJ, Brown GF. Survival of infective larvae of nematode parasites of cattle during drought. Vet Parasitol 1984;14:143–52.
[44] Gibbs HC. Relative importance of winter survival of larval nematodes in pasture and infected carrier calves in a study of parasitic gastroenteritis in calves. Am J Vet Res 1979; 40(2):227–31.
[45] Stuedemann JA, Kaplan RM, Ciordia H, et al. Bermudagrass management in the Southern Piedmont USA V: Gastrointestinal parasite control in cattle. Vet Parasitol 2004;126:375–85.
[46] Craig TM. Seasonal transmission of bovine gastrointestinal nematodes in the Texas Gulf Coast. JAVMA 1979;174:844–7.
[47] Williams JC, Corwin RM, Craig TM, et al. Control strategies for nematodiasis in cattle. Vet Clin North Am Food Anim Pract 1986;2(2):247–60.
[48] Prichard RK. Anthelmintics and control. Vet Parasitol 1988;27:97–109.
[49] Ciordia H. Occurrence of gastrointestinal parasites in Georgia cattle. Am J Vet Res 1975;36: 457–61.
[50] Yazwinski TA, Gibbs HC. Survey of helminth infections in Maine dairy cattle. Am J Vet Res 1975;36:1677–82.
[51] Gibbs HC. The epidemiology of bovine ostertagiasis in the north temperate regions of North America. Vet Parasitol 1988;27:39–47.
[52] Baker NF, Fisk RA. Seasonal occurrence of infective nematode larvae in California Sierra foothill pastures grazed by cattle. Am J Vet Res 1986;47(8):1680–5.
[53] Williams JC, Knox JW, Baumann BA, et al. Seasonal changes of gastrointestinal nematode populations in yearling beef cattle in Louisiana with emphasis on prevalence of inhibition in *Ostertagia ostertagi*. Int J Parasitol 1983;13(2):133–43.
[54] Stromberg BE, Corwin RM. Epizootiology of *Ostertagia osteragi* in cow-calf production systems in the American Midwest. Vet Parasitol 1993;46:297–302.
[55] Southcott WH, Barger IA. Control of nematode parasites by grazing management Part 2. Decontamination of sheep and cattle pastures by varying periods of grazing with the alternative host. Int J Parasitol 1975;5:45–8.
[56] Barger IA, Southcott WH. Control of nematode parasites by grazing management Part I. Decontamination of cattle pastures by grazing with sheep. Int J Parasitol 1975;5:39–44.
[57] Jordan HE, Phillips WA, Morrison RD, et al. A 3-year study of continuous mixed grazing of cattle and sheep: parasitism of offspring. Int J Parasitol 1988;18(6):779–84.
[58] Armour J. The influence of host immunity on the epidemiology of trichostrongyle infections in cattle. Vet Parasitol 1989;32:5–19.
[59] Claerbout E, Dorny P, Vercruysse J, et al. Effects of preventative anthelmintic treatment on acquired resistance to gastrointestinal nematodes in naturally infected cattle. Vet Parasitol 1998;76:287–303.
[60] Ciordia H, Stuedemann JA, Wilkinson SR, et al. Effects of a once-daily suckling program on gastrointestinal parasitism in Angus cows and calves. Am J Vet Res 1985;46:566–9.
[61] Satrija F, Nansen P, Christensen CM. *Ostertagia ostertagi* in neonatal calves: establishment of infection in ruminating and non-ruminating calves. Res Vet Sci 1991;51:344–6.
[62] Gasbarre LC, Leighton EA, Davies CJ. Genetic control of immunity to gastrointestinal nematodes of cattle. Vet Parasitol 1990;37:257–72.
[63] Gibbs HC. The effects of subclinical disease on bovine gastrointestinal nematodiasis. Comped Contin Educ Pract Vet 1992;14(5):669–77.
[64] Newton SE, Munn EA. The development of vaccines against gastrointestinal nematode parasites, particularly *Haemonchus contortus*. Parasitol Today 1999;15(3):116–22.
[65] Barger IA. Influence of sex and reproductive status on susceptibility of ruminants to nematode parasitism. Int J Parasitol 1993;23:463–9.
[66] Borgsteed FHM. Observation on the post-parturient rise of nematode egg-output in cattle. Vet Parasitol 1978;4:385–91.

[67] Connan RM. Effect of lactation on the immune response to gastrointestinal nematodes. Vet Rec 1976;99:476–7.
[68] Leighton EA, Murrell KD, Gasbarre LC. Evidence for genetic control of nematode egg-shedding rates in calves. J Parasitol 1989;75(4):498–504.
[69] Kloosterman A, Albers GAA, van den Brink R. Genetic variation among calves in resistance to nematode parasites. Vet Parasitol 1978;4:353–68.
[70] Williams JC, Knox JW, Barras SA, et al. Effects of ivermectin and fenbendazole in strategic treatment of gastrointestinal nematode infections in cattle. Am J Vet Res 1990;51(12): 2034–43.
[71] Fincher M, Hubbell D, Tucker C, et al. Current and subsequent season effects of parasite control in Arkansas stocker calves. In: Johnson ZB, Kellogg DW, editors. Arkansas Animal Science Department Report. AR Agri Exp Station Research Series 478; 2000. p. 7–9.
[72] Lanusse CE, Pritchard RK. Relationship between pharmacological properties and clinical efficacy of ruminant anthelmintics. Vet Parasitol 1993;49:123–58.
[73] Laffont CM, Alvinerie M, Bousquet-Mélou A, et al. Licking behaviour and environmental contamination arising from pour-on ivermectin for cattle. Int J Parasitol 2001;31:1687–92.
[74] Bousquet-Mélou A, Mercadier S, Alvinerie M, et al. Endectocide exchanges between grazing cattle after pour-on administration of doramectin, ivermectin, and moxidectin. Int J Parasitol 2004;34:1299–307.
[75] Sallovitz J, Lifshitz A, Imperiale F, et al. Breed differences on the plasma availability of moxidectin administered pour-on to calves. Vet J 2002;164:47–53.
[76] Barger IA. Control by management. Vet Parasitol 1997;72:493–506.
[77] Gasbarre LC, Smith LL. Anthelmintic resistance in cattle nematodes—what do we need to know. In: Proceedings of the 50th Annual Meeting of the American Association of Veterinary Parasitologists. Minneapolis, (MN): 2005; Abstract 38.
[78] Coles GC, Jackson F, Pomroy WE, et al. The detection of anthelmintic resistance in nematodes of veterinary importance. Vet Parasitol 2006;136:167–85.
[79] Coles GC. Cattle nematodes resistant to anthelmintics: why so few cases. Vet Res 2002;33: 481–9.
[80] Gasbarre LC, Smith LL, Pillit PA. Identification of cattle nematode parasites resistant to multiple classes of anthelmintics in a commercial cattle population in the US. In: Proceedings of the 50th Annual Meeting of the American Association of Veterinary Parasitologists. Minneapolis, (MN): 2005; Abstract 46.
[81] Geary TG. Ivermectin 20 years on: maturation of a wonder drug. Trends Parasitol 2005; 21(11):530–2.
[82] Lifschitz A, Sallovitz J, Imperiale F, et al. Pharmacokinetic evaluation of four ivermectin generic formulations in calves. Vet Parasitol 2004;119:247–57.
[83] Yazwinski TA, Tucker CA, Hornsby JA, et al. A field trial evaluation of several commercial ivermectin pour-on products in cattle. Arkansas Cattle Business 2004;40(9):44–6.
[84] Wolstenholme AJ, Fairweather I, Prichard R, et al. Drug resistance in veterinary helminths. Trends Parasitol 2004;20(10):469–76.

ELSEVIER
SAUNDERS

Vet Clin Food Anim
22 (2006) 529–541

VETERINARY
CLINICS
Food Animal Practice

Gastrointestinal Nematodes of Small Ruminants: Life Cycle, Anthelmintics, and Diagnosis

Anne M. Zajac, DVM, PhD

Department of Biomedical Sciences and Pathobiology, Virginia/Maryland Regional College of Veterinary Medicine, Virginia Tech, Duckpond Drive, Blacksburg VA 24061-0442, USA

Gastrointestinal nematodes (GIN) infect small ruminants throughout North America and are an important cause of disease and production loss. In the United States in 2001, 74% of sheep producers surveyed indicated that they suspected or confirmed disease caused by stomach and intestinal worms in their animals in the previous 3 years. This high percentage made parasitism the most reported disease category [1]. The GIN of greatest importance in small ruminants are members of the nematode order Strongylida and most belong to the superfamily Trichostrongyloidea. All grazing sheep and goats are infected with a community of these strongylid nematodes whose combined clinical effect is the condition known as parasitic gastroenteritis, or PGE. These parasites are the focus of this article. Basic knowledge of the biology of these organisms is increasingly important for veterinarians and producers designing alternative control strategies in the face of mounting levels of anthelmintic resistance (see article by T. Craig elsewhere in this issue).

Other nematodes belonging to different taxonomic orders also commonly parasitize the small and large bowel of sheep and goats. These nematodes include *Aoncotheca* (formerly called *Capillaria*), *Strongyloides* (small intestine), and *Skrjabinema* and *Trichuris* (large intestine). These parasites are not considered important pathogens and cause disease only in rare circumstances. The presence of their eggs in fecal examinations usually is considered incidental and most will probably be affected by anthelmintics used for more important species.

E-mail address: azajac@vt.edu

0749-0720/06/$ - see front matter
doi:10.1016/j.cvfa.2006.07.006

Important strongylid species

Although all grazing sheep and goats are infected with GIN, low worm burdens usually have little impact on animal health. As worm numbers increase, subclinical effects in the form of reduced weight gain and decreased appetite occur. With heavier worm burdens clinical signs, including weight loss, diarrhea, anemia, and bottle jaw, will develop.

The most important of the strongylid nematodes, not only in the United States but also in many countries around the world, is *Haemonchus contortus*, the barber pole or wireworm. *H contortus* adults are abomasal parasites of small ruminants. Female *H contortus* reach about 3 cm in length, making this species one of the largest of the strongylid nematodes of ruminants. During necropsy, *H contortus* and its distinctive barber pole appearance are not difficult to see in abomasal contents [2].

Haemonchus is one of the most prolific nematodes. A female worm may produce thousands of eggs each day and larvae on pastures can accumulate rapidly during the grazing season in regions where this species predominates. The prepatent period (length of time elapsing between infection of the host and parasite maturity) of *Haemonchus* is about 17 to 21 days [2]. Adult worms are short lived, surviving in the host for only a few months [3].

H contortus has great pathogenic potential because fourth-stage larvae and adults feed on host blood and high parasite numbers can cause fatal anemia. Unlike many other parasites of the gastrointestinal (GI) tract, *H contortus* is not a primary cause of diarrhea [4]. Consequently, its effects on a flock or herd are often insidious because routine observation of animals may not reveal the extent of infection and owners may not appreciate that disease is present until deaths occur. Haemonchosis and PGE in general occur most often in young, nonimmune animals, adult animals whose immunity has been compromised, or in sheep or goats exposed to very high levels of infection. Although other trichostrongylid nematodes can add to the burden of parasitism in small ruminants, *H contortus* is the primary cause of losses because of GIN in much of the United States [5].

A second important trichostrongylid nematode that contributes to PGE in the United States is *Teladorsagia circumcincta* (formerly *Ostertagia circumcincta*). Like *H contortus*, *T circumcincta* is a parasite of the abomasum. Unlike *H contortus*, however, *T circumcincta* does not feed primarily on blood nor are the females as prolific. Following infection, *T circumcincta* larvae spend a variable period of time developing in the abomasal gastric glands. These larvae cause changes in the glands that lead to formation of visible nodules on the mucosal surface of the abomasum [2]. In heavy infections, sheep or goats may develop diarrhea, anemia, or hypoproteinemia, and in severe cases death can occur. More commonly, moderate infections of *T circumcincta* could contribute to PGE with signs including diarrhea and poor weight gain or weight loss. *T circumcincta* is a smaller parasite than *H contortus* (females are ~1 cm long) [2]. On necropsy of infected animals the abomasal nodules produced by larvae can be seen, but the worms themselves are difficult to find in the abomasal contents and are often missed. The prepatent period of this parasite is approximately 3 weeks and, like *Haemonchus*, the life span of adult worms is only a few months [4]. Although *T circumcincta* is found throughout the United States it does not have the pathogenic importance of *H contortus*.

Trichostrongylus is a third common genus of trichostrongylid nematode that causes disease in heavy infections, but more often is a contributor to PGE in the United States. Several species of *Trichostrongylus* infect small ruminants, including *T axei*, an abomasal parasite, and *T colubriformis* and *T vitrinus*, which are found in the small intestine. These small worms (<1 cm) [2] are not readily visible in abomasal and intestinal contents and infection will only be detected if contents are removed and examined closely. Adult *Trichostrongylus* are longer lived than *Teladorsagia* and *Haemonchus* adults and can survive over winter as adults in the host [3]. Heavy burdens of *Trichostrongylus* can cause severe diarrhea (called "black scours"), weight loss, and death [6]. Recently two cases of human infection with *Trichostrongylus* were reported from Australia. Infected individuals used fresh goat manure as fertilizer for vegetables that were consumed raw [7]. Similar cases could occur in the United States as the popularity of diversified small farms increases.

Other strongylid species

Cooperia curticei, *Nematodirus spathiger*, and *N filicollis* are common parasites of the small intestine of sheep and goats, as is *Oesophagostomum venulosum* in the large bowel. *Bunostomum trigonocephalum* and *Chabertia ovina* are less common parasites of the small intestine and large intestine, respectively. These species are rarely pathogenic alone, but may contribute to PGE [8]. *Nematodirus battus*, which causes severe diarrhea in lambs in some European countries, was identified in the United States in sheep and llamas for the first time in the 1980s in the Pacific Northwest and subsequently was found in a national survey of sheep in Washington, Maryland, New York, and Vermont [9]. The discovery of the parasite aroused concern that it could become an important pathogen in North America. Disease problems associated with the parasite have not developed to date, however.

Host specificity

Mixed or alternate grazing with cattle or horses typically is recommended as a component of small ruminant integrated parasite control programs and producers are often concerned about the risk for cross-infection. Cattle are infected by the same genera of parasites as small ruminants, but usually have their own strains or species. In general, the strongylid species of small ruminants do not successfully infect horses or cattle and larvae are killed when ingested by those host species. Two exceptions to this generalization should be noted. Calves may be susceptible to *H contortus* infections and should not be exposed to pastures heavily contaminated with this parasite. Similarly, sheep can become infected with *H placei*, the bovine *Haemonchus* species, although this parasite is not a major pathogen in the United States [10]. Second, *T axei* has wider host specificity than most members of this group of worms and successfully infects cattle and horses. In reality, however, *T axei* infections in the United States usually are minor and the parasite has not become a clinical problem for mixed or alternate grazing systems [5].

Producers often are interested to know if small ruminant nematodes can infect white-tailed deer, because deer are now common in much of the United States and frequently invade small ruminant pastures. Deer have been infected successfully with *H contortus* of sheep origin experimentally [11], although they probably do not play a large role in the epidemiology of the parasite in small ruminants.

Life cycle

The same life cycle generally applies to all of the economically important strongylid parasites of small ruminants in the United States. In this simple cycle, adult female parasites in the abomasum or intestines produce eggs that are passed in the manure. Development occurs within the fecal mass, which provides some protection from environmental conditions. A first-stage larva is formed that hatches out of the egg. After hatching, larvae feed on bacteria and undergo two molts to reach the infective third larval stage (L3). Third-stage larvae make their way out of the fecal material and onto the forage where they are ingested by sheep and goats [2].

Nematodirus spp are an exception to the life cycle described above. The L3 develops inside the egg before hatching occurs. In the case of *N battus*, hatching is stimulated by a period of low temperature followed by higher temperature, leading to the synchronous appearance of larvae in the northern European environments where the parasite can be a serious pathogen. The concentrated exposure to L3 intensifies the pathogenic effects of this parasite. In the Pacific Northwest, however, transmission of *N battus* may occur year round, which may be a factor in the decreased pathogenicity of *N battus* seen in the United States [12].

Strongylid larva biology

The fortunes of strongylid larvae in the microenvironment of the fecal pellets and on herbage ultimately determine whether or not a producer battles parasitic disease. For their part, the parasites struggle against variable environmental conditions, first to develop to the infective stage, second to move successfully from the feces to the herbage where they can be ingested by the host, and finally to survive long enough to infect the host. Not all the species have the same environmental preferences and the distribution and importance of species therefore varies across the United States. Understanding the biology of the immature parasites is useful in predicting parasite distribution and formulating integrated parasite control programs.

In general, development of trichostrongylid larvae occurs in a temperature range of approximately 10°C to 36°C (50°F–96°F). *H contortus* is the predominant GIN of small ruminants in the United States, not only because of its pathogenicity but also because this prolific parasite finds the climate in a large part of the country highly favorable for development and survival of its infective larvae [2]. *H contortus* develops most successfully in warm wet climates and does not tolerate cold temperatures well. The southeastern United States in particular, with its hot, humid summers and long grazing season, is well suited to *H contortus* [13–15]. Even in northeastern and midwestern states, summer grazing season conditions provide an appropriate environment for *H contortus* development and the parasite is important in these areas also [8,16–18], although the period of transmission is shorter than in southern states. Optimum conditions for transmission of *H contortus* were found from May through September in Urbana, Illinois, whereas in Columbus, Georgia optimum conditions were present from mid-March to mid-October [19]. Even within broad environmental preferences for each species, there is evidence of local adaptation. Eggs of a strain of *H contortus* from England, with its cooler summer temperatures, hatched at lower temperatures than *H contortus* strains from Kentucky and New York [20].

Teladorsagia and *Trichostrongylus* spp are found throughout the United States but their transmission seasons are different from those of *Haemonchus* because these species are more successful in cooler, drier conditions. In Illinois, peak conditions for *Trichostrongylus* and *Teladorsagia* transmission occurred in two periods, from March to June and September to November. In Georgia they occurred from October to almost May [19]. In both states conditions for transmission were not favorable in hot summer weather. These two genera replace *Haemonchus* in importance only in the western states where cold winters and dry summers reduce the success of *H contortus* [21]. When developing eggs of *Haemonchus* and *Teladorsagia* isolated in Washington state were experimentally exposed to a 15-hour period of −18°C, it was found that whereas >87% of *T circumcincta* eggs were subsequently able to hatch, <4% of *H contortus* eggs hatched [22]. Similarly, when L3 of the two species were exposed to −18°C for 5 hours, the viability of *H contortus* L3 declined to <5% whereas *T circumcincta* L3 viability was 85% [23].

The arid summers in many western states also reduce transmission rates of most GIN and PGE is generally less important than in the eastern United States [21]. For example, few larvae appear to survive the dry winters of western Texas [24]. Even *Haemonchus* can become an important parasite in dry regions where irrigation occurs, however. In a study comparing irrigated with nonirrigated pasture in Utah, conditions were suitable for transmission of *Haemonchus* on irrigated pasture during 5 of the 6 months of the experiment. In contrast, conditions were never suitable for transmission on the nonirrigated pasture during the study [25].

The length of time required for development to the L3 stage varies with temperature. The minimum length of time required for the development of *H contortus* larvae is about 3 to 4 days [2], and rapid turnover of eggs into larvae can occur in hot summer weather. In contrast, eggs deposited in cool spring weather develop more slowly and may require several months to become L3. As a result, cool spring pastures in more northern states may not carry a substantial burden of infective larvae until late spring or early summer [26].

Once infective larvae have formed, they must leave the fecal pellet and migrate onto forage. Rain is important in releasing larvae from the manure onto the herbage. During dry weather, larvae will be retained in the manure pellets. With the next rain there will be a burst of larval release. Producers may see an outbreak of parasitic disease a few weeks after the end of a period of drought when animals are exposed to large numbers of newly available L3 [5].

L3 can migrate laterally and vertically in films of moisture on herbage. The ability of larvae to migrate is affected by air temperature, soil moisture, and relative humidity [27]. *H contortus* larvae were able to migrate up to 90 cm away from fecal pellets, but most remain within about 10 cm of the feces. In hot, dry weather, when no moisture is on the grass, larvae are unable to migrate on the herbage [28]. The activity of dung beetles and earthworms breaks up fecal material and reduces the number of L3 by exposing more susceptible first- and second-stage larvae to desiccation and ultraviolet light [29]. Forage type also seems to influence migration of larvae on pastures, which may be a result of differences in temperature and humidity in stands of different forages or the ease with which the moisture film required by L3 develops on leaves [30].

The length of time that infective larvae can survive on the pasture is important for pasture management programs that aim to control parasitism. Nematodes are covered by a tough semipermeable outer layer called the cuticle. The cuticle is replaced with each molt, but the L3 larva retains the cuticle of the second-stage larva as a sheath. Although the sheath gives these larvae greater resistance to environmental conditions, it also prevents them from feeding. Once an L3 uses its stored metabolic reserves it dies. Consequently, the best conditions for survival of infective larvae are cool, dry weather, because dry weather reduces movement of the larvae [10]. Cool, moist weather also supports survival of L3 for many months. L3 survives for much shorter periods in hot weather. In the temperate portions of the United States, a pasture that has been grazed by sheep or goats must be rested for 6 months during cool weather to be considered safe. In hot weather, most larvae may be cleared from pasture in 3 months [5].

Hypobiosis

The epidemiology of important species of GIN is also strongly influenced by aspects of host–parasite biology after infection occurs. Larvae of important GIN are able to undergo a period of arrested development (hypobiosis) in the host. Following infection, larvae may become metabolically inactive for a period that may last several months and then resume development. Although the immune status of the host also has an influence on rates of hypobiosis, the greatest proportion of larvae usually arrest at times of the year when conditions in the environment are least favorable for development and survival of eggs and larvae [31]. In areas with cold winters, *Haemonchus* survives the winter months primarily as arrested larvae. In tracer lambs in Ohio, Maine, Virginia, and Pennsylvania more than 80% of *Haemonchus* and some other GIN were present as arrested larvae in winter [16,32]. Even without anthelmintic treatment in states with cold winters, *Haemonchus* problems resolve at the end of the grazing season because most newly ingested larvae become arrested in the host. Consequently, as existing adult worms die they are not immediately replaced. Also, eggs that are shed at the end of the grazing season are unlikely to develop or develop slowly, preventing further buildup of L3 on pasture. Where winters are very mild, hypobiosis seems to be less important in the epidemiology of parasite transmission. In Louisiana, levels of hypobiotic larvae were never substantial in tracer lambs followed throughout the year, although the highest proportion of hypobiotic larvae tended to be in the fall [15].

In areas where winter arrest of parasite larvae occurs, emergence and development of adult worms in late winter and spring are followed by an increase in fecal eggs counts. The rise in egg counts is magnified in periparturient animals by a relaxation of immunity that increases survival and egg production in existing parasites and also increases susceptibility to further infection. The periparturient egg rise (PPR) can make an important contribution to L3 populations on pastures as young, susceptible animals begin grazing [33]. The PPR is well documented in sheep, but may not be as important epidemiologically in goats.

Anthelmintics

Since the advent in the 1960s of modern broad-spectrum anthelmintics with wide safety margins producers have relied on dewormers for control of GIN in the United States. In the southeastern United States, where *H contortus* causes substantial losses, frequent treatments were used (and recommended to producers) throughout the grazing season in suppressive anthelmintic programs that kept egg production and pasture contamination at low levels. The outcome of this intensive anthelmintic use is widespread resistance in GIN nematode populations, especially in *H contortus* [5]. For most producers, parasite control continues to include treatments with anthelmintic drugs, but any veterinarian working with small ruminant producers must stress the importance of alternative methods of parasite control that can be used in combination with anthelmintics. A further incentive for veterinarians to look beyond anthelmintic control programs is the increased interest of producers in sustainable and organic production practices.

All of the approved available anthelmintics for sheep or goats in the United States fall into one of three major drug groups: the benzimidazoles, the cholinergic agonists, and the macrocyclic lactones. When a population of worms becomes resistant to one member of a drug group, it effectively becomes resistant to the other members of the group. The following products are currently approved for use in sheep and goats in the United States:

Benzimidazoles (BZDs). Albendazole (ABZ) and fenbendazole (FBZ) are the BZD products marketed in the United States for small ruminants. At this time ABZ is approved for use in sheep and FBZ for use in goats. The primary mode of action of benzimidazoles is to inhibit microtubule formation [6]. Albendazole is approved for use in sheep at a dose rate of 7.5 mg/kg. Because ABZ has embryotoxic effects at 11 mg/kg in early pregnancy it is contraindicated for use in the first 30 days of gestation. Based on the pharmacokinetics of this drug group in small ruminants, several techniques have been recommended to maximize drug efficacy in the host. Withholding feed from sheep or goats 12 to 24 hours before treatment slows passage of the drug through the GI tract and improves absorption. It is also important to place BZD drenches in the back of the mouth to avoid stimulating closure of the esophageal groove. Finally, goats metabolize these drugs differently than sheep and require higher doses than sheep. Additional information on best practices for use of these and other anthelmintics is available at the website of the Southern Consortium for Small Ruminant Parasite Control: http://www.scsrpc.org/SCSRPC/Files/Files/Misc/DRENSHIN.PDF.

Macrocyclic lactones. The macrocyclic lactones include two products approved for oral use in sheep: ivermectin (0.2 mg/kg) and moxidectin (0.2 mg/kg). Other macrolides approved for use in cattle in the United States are eprinomectin and doramectin. The macrocyclic lactones are an extremely powerful group of anthelmintics with activity against nematodes and arthropods. The drugs in this group interfere with chloride channel neurotransmission [6]. Macrocyclic lactones have been used extensively by small ruminant producers and widespread resistance to the group is seen in *H contortus* and other strongylids in the Southeast [34]. In general these products are extremely safe, although there are anecdotal reports of moxidectin toxicity in very young animals. Although these products are not approved for goats they have been widely adopted by producers and inappropriate use may have contributed to the rapid growth in resistant parasites. Because of differences in metabolism, goats should be given a higher dose of ivermectin than sheep. Currently, ivermectin is the only anthelmintic approved for limited use in nonslaughter organically raised sheep in the United States, although continued use of the product is under consideration by the National Organic Standards Board [35].

Nicotinic anthelmintics. This group of anthelmintics includes levamisole, pyrantel, and morantel. All work on the parasite nervous system as nicotinic agonists and cause paralysis of nematodes [6]. Although levamisole is chemically different from pyrantel and morantel, they share the same mode of action and resistance to one compound is expected to cause resistance to other members of the group. Levamisole is marketed as a soluble powder for sheep and morantel is approved for use as a feed additive for goats.

Diagnosis of gastrointestinal strongylid parasites

The primary laboratory test used for the diagnosis of strongylid nematodes is a fecal flotation procedure for detection of the eggs of the parasites. Strongylid nematode genera produce eggs that are similar in appearance and cannot be easily discriminated (Fig. 1). In fecal samples they are all identified in general terms as strongylid or trichostrongylid eggs. To identify the genera of these nematodes, fecal culture and identification of L3 larvae are required. The exception in the United States is eggs of *Nematodirus* spp (and *Marshallagia*, a genus found in the western United States). These eggs are much larger and contain distinctive dark cells (Fig. 2) [36].

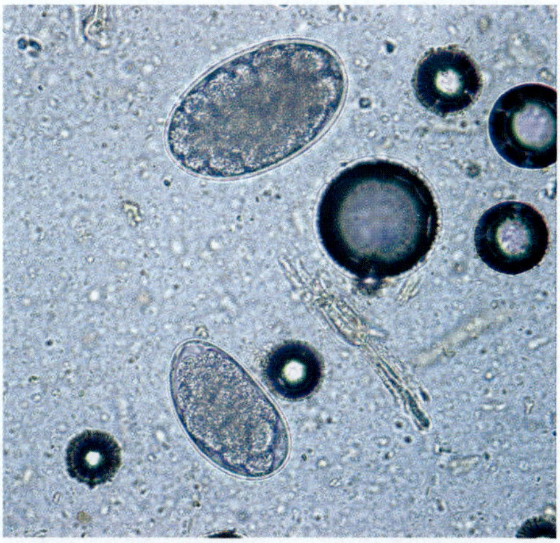

Fig. 1. Strongylid eggs in feces of a sheep. These eggs range in size from approximately 65 to 100 μm in length. Genus identification cannot accurately and consistently be made from observation of eggs in fecal examinations.

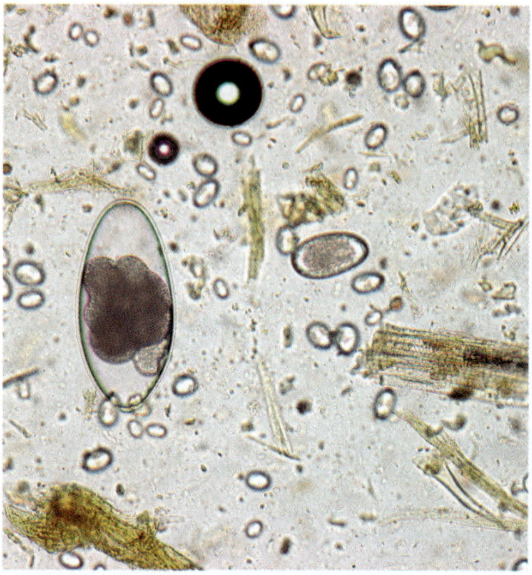

Fig. 2. Egg of *Nematodirus* in feces of a sheep. This large egg (~150–250 μm) is easily differentiated from ordinary strongylid eggs by its large size and large dark cells.

Because virtually all grazing small ruminants are infected with some gastrointestinal nematodes, a simple flotation procedure that simply detects the presence of strongylid parasites is of limited value. The most useful herd or flock test is a quantitative egg-counting technique. Fecal egg counts can be used to evaluate the efficacy of parasite control programs, monitor levels of potential pasture contamination, and monitor drug efficacy. Fecal egg counts can also be used in young animals as a tool for genetic selection for resistance to GIN [36,37]. Because most eggs of strongylid nematodes cannot be differentiated consistently, egg counting techniques are valuable as herd tools but of limited use for diagnosis of disease in individual animals. Individual fecal egg counts can be influenced by the consistency of the feces, prolificacy of species and stages of parasite present, and recent anthelmintic use.

Because small ruminants often have egg counts in excess of several hundred eggs per gram of feces, the most practical quantitative technique is the Modified McMaster Test. This test requires the use of a special counting chamber (available in the United States from Chalex Corporation, Issaquah WA, www.vetslides.com). McMaster slides are plastic and can last for many years with simple care. Many sources provide instructions for the Modified McMaster Test and each is slightly different (for examples see: RVC/FAO Guide to Veterinary Diagnostic Parasitology, http://www.fao.org/ag/againfo/resources/documents/Parasitology/EggCount/Purpose.htm; the webpage of the Southeastern Consortium for Small Ruminant Parasite Control, www.scsrpc.org; the webpage of the E[Kika] De La Garza Institute for

Goat Research, http://www2.luresext.edu/goats/library/fec4.html; the article by Ballweber, elsewhere in this issue; or [36]). The most important thing about the test is that whatever technique is used, it must be used consistently so that comparisons over time are possible.

Fecal samples collected for analysis should be either from the rectum or from the ground immediately after passage from the animal. Samples that will be sent to a diagnostic laboratory should be wrapped in foil or plastic wrap and placed in zip-lock bags with the air expressed from the bag. Keeping oxygen levels low prevents normal development of eggs. Samples processed in this way can be sent by regular mail for analysis. Development can also be slowed, but not stopped, by placing samples in the refrigerator. Eggs will eventually develop and hatch, especially those of the more cold-tolerant genera like *Trichostrongylus* and *Teladorsagia*. A solution of 10% formalin can be added to preserve fecal samples for long periods. Fecal samples should not be frozen because eggs will be killed.

For flock or herd monitoring, samples should be collected from a proportion of animals representing all age, gender, and reproductive categories. It is preferable to analyze samples from individual animals. The use of pooled samples has been controversial because pools may not contain animals shedding high numbers of parasite eggs that are responsible for a significant proportion of pasture contamination. Conversely, if those animals are included, results of a pooled sample will indicate that most animals are shedding more parasite eggs than they actually are. In situations in which composite samples are the only practical means of monitoring a flock or herd, however, several composites should be formed by combining samples within reproductive and age groups.

The Modified McMaster Test can also be used in a fecal egg count reduction test (FECRT) to test anthelmintic efficacy. In the face of increasing anthelmintic resistance, practitioners can offer clients a valuable service by evaluating whether the drugs they are using are still effective. To conduct an FECRT, 10 to 15 animals should be selected as an untreated control group and a similar number for each drug to be tested. All the animals in the test should have at least 150 eggs/g of feces and may need to be tested before the trial if there is uncertainty about the level of eggs in the feces. Animals in the test group must be treated individually. The correct dose of the drug must be given either based on individual animal weights or all animals treated with the dose accurately determined for the heaviest animal in the group. Fecal samples should be collected from animals in the treatment and control groups 10 to 14 days later and fecal egg counts performed. The percentage reduction in fecal egg counts is based on the formula: % reduction = 100 (1 − [TM/CM]) where TM is the mean egg count of the treated group and CM is the mean egg count of the untreated control group [38].

For practical purposes, in small ruminants a fecal egg count reduction of less than 90% suggests that resistant worms may be present. The lower the egg count reduction the higher the proportion of resistant worms in the population. For example, a fecal egg count reduction of 40% indicates a higher proportion of resistant worms than a reduction of 80%.

References

[1] NAHMS. Sheep 2001 Part II: Reference of Sheep Health in the United States 2001. 2003. Available at: http://www.aphis.usda.gov/vs/ceah/ncahs/nahms/sheep/sheep01/sheep01Pt2.pdf)\. Accessed May 1, 2006.

[2] Levine N. Trichostrongyles. In: Nematode parasites of domestic animals and of man. Minneapolis: Burgess Publishing Company; 1980. p. 135–221.

[3] Courtney CH, Parker CF, McClure KE, et al. Population dynamics of *Haemonchus contortus* and *Trichostrongylus* spp in sheep. Int J Parasitol 1983;13:557–60.

[4] Soulsby EJL. Nematodes of the gastrointestinal tract. In: Textbook of veterinary clinical parasitology. Vol. 1: Helminths. Philadelphia: F. A. Davis Company; 1965. p. 414–44.

[5] Fleming S, Craig T, Kaplan RM, et al. Anthelmintic resistance of gastrointestinal parasites in small ruminants. J Vet Intern Med 2006;20:435–44.

[6] Bowman DD. Helminths. In: Georgi's parasitology for veterinarians. 8th edition. St. Louis: Saunders; 1999. p. 115–244.

[7] Ralph A, O'Sullivan MVN, Sangster NC, et al. Abdominal pain and eosinophilia in suburban goat keepers. Med J Aust 2006;184:467–9.

[8] Herd RP. Epidemiology and control of gastrointestinal nematodes and cestodes in small ruminants: Northern United States. Vet Clin N Amer Food Anim Prac 1986;2:367–72.

[9] Zimmerman GL, Hoberg EP, Rickard LG, et al. Broadened geographic range and periods of transmission for *Nematodirus battus* in the United States. Proc US Anim Health Assoc 1986; 90:404–12.

[10] Barger IA. The role of epidemiological knowledge and grazing management for helminth control in small ruminants. Int J Parasitol 1999;29:41–7.

[11] Foreyt W, Trainer DO. Experimental haemonchosis in white-tailed deer. J Wild Dis 1970;6: 35–42.

[12] Rickard LG, Hoberg E, Zimmerman GL, et al. Late fall transmission of *Nematodirus battus* (Nematoda:Trichostrongyloidea) in Western Oregon. J Parasitol 1987;73:244–7.

[13] Craig T. Epidemiology and control of gastrointestinal nematodes and cestodes in small ruminants: Southern United States. Vet Clin N Amer Food Anim Prac 1986;2:367–72.

[14] Amarante AFT, Craig TM, Ramsey WS, et al. Comparison of naturally acquired parasite burdens among Florida Native, Rambouillet and crossbreed ewes. Vet Parasitol 1999;85: 61–9.

[15] Miller JE, Bahirathan M, Lemarie SL, et al. Epidemiology of gastrointestinal nematode parasitism in Suffolk and Gulf Coast Native sheep with special emphasis on relative susceptibility to *Haemonchus contortus* infection. Vet Parasitol 1998;74:55–74.

[16] Coyne MJ, Smith G, Johnstone C. Fecundity of gastrointestinal trichostrongylid nematodes of sheep in the field. Am J Vet Res 1991;52:1182–8.

[17] Aaylew L, Gibbs HC. Seasonal fluctuations of nematode populations in breeding ewes and lambs. Can J Comp Med 1973;37:79–89.

[18] Levine ND, Clark DT, Bradley RE, et al. Relationship of pasture rotation to acquisition of gastrointestinal nematodes in sheep. Am J Vet Res 1975;36:1459–64.

[19] Levine ND. Weather, climate and the bionomics of ruminant nematode larvae. Adv Vet Sci 1963;8:215–61.

[20] Crofton HD, Whitlock JH, Glazer RA. Ecology and biological plasticity of sheep nematodes. II. Genetic X environmental plasticity in *Haemonchus contortus* (Rud. 1803). Cornell Vet 1965;55:251–9.

[21] Wescott RB. Epidemiology and control of nematodes and cestodes in small ruminants: Western states. Vet Clin N Amer: Food Anim Prac 1986;2:363–6.
[22] Jasmer DP, Wescott RB, Crane JW. Influence of cold temperatures upon development and survival of eggs of Washington isolates of *Haemonchus contortus* and *Ostertagia circumcincta*. Proc Helminthol Soc Wash 1986;53:244–7.
[23] Jasmer DP, Wescott RB, Crane JW. Survival of third-stage larvae of Washington isolates of *Haemonchus contortus* and *Ostertagia circumcincta*. Proc Helminthol Soc Wash 1987;54: 48–52.
[24] Craig T, Miller D. Controlling internal parasites. Ranch Magazine 1989:14–20.
[25] Bullick GR, Andersen FL. Effect of irrigation on survival of third-stage *Haemonchus contortus* larvae (Nematoda: Trichostrongylidae). Great Basin Nat 1978;38:369–78.
[26] Herd RP. A practical approach to parasite control in sheep in the Northern United States. Comp Cont Ed Prac Vet 1984;6:S67–73.
[27] Krecek RC, Hartman R, Groeneveld HT, et al. Microclimatic effect on vertical migration of *Haemonchus contortus* and *Haemonchus placei* third-stage larvae on irrigated Kikuyu pasture. Onderstepoort J Vet Res 1995;62:117–22.
[28] Skinner WD, Todd KS. Lateral migration of *Haemonchus contortus* larvae on pasture. Am J Vet Res 1980;41:395–8.
[29] Stromberg BE. Environmental factors influencing transmission. Vet Parasitol 1997;72: 247–64.
[30] Niezen JH, Charleston WAG, Hodgson J, et al. Effect of plant species on the larvae of gastrointestinal nematodes which parasitize sheep. Int J Parasitol 1998;28:791–803.
[31] Eysker M. Some aspects of inhibited development of trichostrongylids in ruminants. Vet Parasitol 1997;72:265–83.
[32] Zajac AM, Moore GA. Treatment and control of gastrointestinal nematodes in sheep. Comp Cont Ed Prac Vet 1993;15:999–1012.
[33] Gibbs HC. Hypobiosis and the periparturient rise in sheep. Vet Clin N Amer: Food Anim Prac 1986;2:345–53.
[34] Mortensen LL, Williamson LH, Terrill TH, et al. Evaluation of prevalence and clinical implications of anthelmintic resistance in gastrointestinal nematodes of goats. JAVMA 2003; 223:495–500.
[35] National Center for Appropriate Technology (NCAT). NCAT's organic livestock workbook. A guide to sustainable allowed practices. 2004. p. 54. Available at: http://attra.ncat.org/attra-pub/summaries/livestockworkbook.html. Accessed May 1, 2006.
[36] Zajac AM, Conboy GA. Fecal Examination for the diagnosis of parasitism. In: Veterinary Clinical Parasitology, 7th edition. Ames: Blackwell Publishing; 2006. p. 3–142.
[37] Pugh DG, Navarre CB. Internal parasite control strategies. Vet Clin N Amer: Food Anim Prac 2001;17:231–45.
[38] Coles GC, Bauer C, Borgsteede FHM, et al. World Association for the Advancement of Veterinary Parasitology (W.A.A.V.P.) methods for the detection of anthelmintic resistance in nematodes of veterinary importance. Vet Parasitol 1992;44:35–44.

ELSEVIER
SAUNDERS

Vet Clin Food Anim
22 (2006) 543–565

VETERINARY
CLINICS
Food Animal Practice

Gastrointestinal Nematode Control Programs with an Emphasis on Cattle

Bert E. Stromberg, PhD[a,*], Louis C. Gasbarre, PhD[b]

[a]*Veterinary and Biomedical Sciences Department, College of Veterinary Medicine, University of Minnesota, 1971 Commonwealth Avenue, St. Paul, MN 55108, USA*
[b]*Bovine Functional Genomics Laboratory, Agricultural Research Service, Building 200, Room 6, BARC-East ARS, United Sates Department of Agriculture, Beltsville, MD 20705, USA*

Control strategies for nematode parasites rely on knowledge of the relationships between the parasites and their hosts. Specifically, these programs are based on identifying crucial points of interaction in the environment provided by the host, including genetics and the immune response, and critical periods in the physical environment in which the eggs and larval stages must develop. When these targets are identified and the interactions understood, cost-effective sustainable programs can be developed using currently available antiparasitic compounds. Resistance to the major classes of anthelmintic compounds requires consideration of new approaches, such as immunity or genetics of the host. Additionally, the efficacy of these compounds can be expanded with combined or concomitant use. Increased study of the use of novel approaches, including fungi, elements such as copper, and plant products, has also occurred. This article explores each of these areas to allow readers to appreciate how various approaches may be developed and incorporated into an effective parasite control program.

Parasite dynamics

Cattle helminths live on the pasture and in their host. The adult worms live and reproduce within the cow, whereas the eggs that the parasites produce pass in the fecal material and contaminate the pasture. The eggs then hatch and develop into the infective stage on the herbage, causing cattle to become

* Corresponding author.
E-mail address: b-stro@umn.edu (B.E. Stromberg).

0749-0720/06/$ - see front matter. Published by Elsevier Inc.
doi:10.1016/j.cvfa.2006.08.003

infected from ingesting infective larvae when grazing. These developing parasites are controlled by two environments: the host and the pasture.

Parasite dynamics on pasture

Cattle intestinal helminths contaminate the pasture with large numbers of eggs. Some worms. such a *Cooperia* spp, are prolific when compared with the less-fecund *Ostertagia ostertagi.* The worms mate and begin to produce eggs that are passed in the fecal material. Pasture contamination, in addition to the impact of worm fecundity, is directly dependent on the stocking rate; more animals in a confined area will deposit more feces and thus more eggs per unit area.

How much parasite contamination accrues over a typical grazing season? Studies have found that the amount of fecal material produced is related to the weight of the animal, whereas the number of times the animal defecates per day is related to the age of animal (cow vs. calf) [1]. The average calf will defecate 6.23 times per day, whereas a cow defecates 8.1 times in 24 hours. The amount of fecal material is directly related to the weight of the animal, and can be calculated using the following equation: pat weight = 0.000285 $W^{1.316}$ (W = body weight). Typically, helminth egg shedding is measured by determining the number of eggs per gram (EPG) of fecal material. If the EPG, age, and weight of the animal are known, the total number of helminth eggs produced in 24 hours can be calculated. This calculation can be extended to the total number produced over any period or the numbers produced by the herd. The pasture contamination of individual animals and the herd provides some insight into the total contamination over a grazing season. A 150-lb calf with an EPG of 100 produces 73,733 eggs every 24 hours, whereas the dam (1400 lb; 18 EPG) produces 360,705 eggs each 24 hours. This output occurs every day of the grazing season. An average cow–calf pair produces approximately 51 million eggs in approximately 3 tons of manure over a typical 5-month grazing season [1].

When the eggs are shed in the fecal material, they must hatch and develop to the infective larval stage within the environment of the fecal pat. When the larvae molt to the third stage, they retain the sheath that provides some protection against environmental factors, particularly desiccation. Under optimal environmental conditions (25°C), Ciordia and Bizzell found that *O ostertagi* eggs will hatch in 12 to 24 hours and develop into the infective L_3 in 5 to 6 days [2]. These investigators also observed that only 30% of the eggs actually developed to the infective stage at 25°C, with even lower developmental success at higher and lower temperatures (5.3% at 32°C and 21.5% at 20°C, respectively). These observations vary; one study reported that *O ostertagi* eggs took up to 42 days to develop at 5°C [3], whereas Ciordia and Bizzell [2] found that the eggs did not develop to the infective stage at this temperature. When trying to infect rabbits with

Trichostronylus axei, Ciordia and colleagues [4] found that viable larvae lost infectivity as the temperature increased.

Temperature seems to drive the developmental process, but development does not proceed without moisture. Levine [5] found that good conditions for transmission of *Haemonchus contortus* and *Trichostrongylus* were approximately 2.5 cm (approximately 1 in) or more of precipitation per month, with temperature ranges from 15°C to 32°C and 6°C to 20°C, respectively. These reported numbers and times for development vary greatly for different climatic regions. The ranges of moisture also seem to be somewhat regional, with good-to-optimal development occurring in 2.6 to 9.4 cm of precipitation in Maryland [6] and 5 to 17 cm in Louisiana [7].

Larvae must move away from the fecal pat and onto the surrounding herbage to be ingested by the ruminant host and continue its life cycle. The availability of nematode larvae to grazing animals depends on moisture [8,9] for providing a water film to allow migration. Krecek and colleagues [10] also found temperature to be an important factor in migration. Tarshis [11] observed that a mixture of trichostrongyle-type larvae migrated as far as 40 cm from the fecal pat in an artificial plot and that this migration differed between grass types, fescue (16 in), red clover (11 in), and oats (8 in). Levine and colleagues [12] found that many of the larvae migrated out onto the herbage or into the thatch (grass mat) and very few were found in the upper portions of the soil. Williams and Bilkovich [13] recovered most of the larvae between 2.5 and 15 cm from the fecal pats. They also observed more larvae on the upper herbage (8 to 16 cm) than on the lower portion (soil to 8 cm). Stromberg [1] observed that few trichostrongyle larvae migrated more than 15 cm from the center of the dung pat (5 cm from the edge) and very few were ever recovered from the soil. He also observed that the numbers of larvae on the herbage were directly related to the number of eggs in the fecal material and the size of the dung pat.

Numerous studies have found that the microclimate at the base of the herbage is very favorable for larval survival and may harbor large numbers of ruminant parasite larvae [14,15]. More recently, Krecek and Murrell [16] described the ability of *O ostertagi* to migrate vertically and laterally through the soil and then back onto the herbage. Some larvae migrated as far as 15 cm down into a primarily sand-based soil and returned to the surface. Grønvold and Høgh-Schmidt [17] found substantial numbers of larvae in the soil beneath their artificial cow pats, but did not report the depth or soil type. It is attractive to postulate that sandy soil may serve as a reservoir of moisture and larvae during periods of dryness.

Moisture also plays a significant role in the movement of larvae away from the dung pat and up onto the grass. Grønvold [18] and Grønvold and Høgh-Schmidt [17] observed that as cow pats dried, the number of active larvae available at the surface decreased, presumably migrating into the pat or being trapped in the crust. When the pat was sprayed with water, the number of larvae on the surface increased and were available for distribution. Using simulated rainfall, they also found that few larvae were dispersed when the drops fell on pats with a dry surface, but that when the surface was moist (watered), a significant number of larvae were transported away from the cow pat. They observed that more than 90% of the larvae were translocated by the splash droplets and only a minor proportion migrated actively in the water film on the herbage. Larvae were found as far as 90 cm (35 in) from the experimental pat.

These infective larvae may survive for days to months, depending on the species and environmental conditions. The ensheathed infective larvae are generally more resistant to pasture conditions than those in the developing stages. Obviously, very few larvae survive the harsh summers in the southern states [13] or harsh winters in the north. However, when larvae are protected by a blanket of snow, an increased number may survive the winter. Stromberg and colleagues [19] found that *O ostertagi* larvae survived on pasture from July through the winter and into the next spring (April), when tracer calves became infected after grazing on the pasture. Experts generally agree that larvae tend to lose infectivity as they age [4], and that fewer parasites are found in cooler temperatures (climate). Although the numbers are dramatically reduced under these harsh conditions, a few parasites survive and continue to provide a source of reinfection.

Fincher [20] showed that dung-burying beetles could substantially reduce the number of *O ostertagi* larvae on experimental plots. Each plot had a different sized beetle population (ie, *Phanaeus spp, Dictotomius* sp). The largest population was able to bury all feces placed on the plot within 96 hours and was able to reduce the pasture larval population by 14.7-fold. The role of dung beetles on natural transmission was also evaluated by placing parasite-free calves on contaminated pastures, each with a different sized dung beetle population. The larger the beetle population, the fewer the worms recovered from the calves [21].

Bergstrom and colleagues [22] found that the smaller coprophagous beetles (eg, *Aphodius, Canthon*) were also highly effective in reducing the number of trichostrongylid eggs, by up to 90% in 5 days. These beetles do not bury the dung but rather ingest a portion of the feces and spread the remaining portion on the herbage. Byran and Kerr [23] reported that pasture populations of helminth larvae were reduced by up to 44%. These authors also observed the relationship among the dung beetle, larval helminths, and rainfall. Increased rainfall increased the pasture larval counts and reduced the beetle populations, indicating that none of these factors works independently. Birds disrupt the fecal pat by feeding on arthropod larvae in the dung. Earthworms also disrupt the fecal pat and cause subsequent desiccation. These factors are all responsible for reducing larvae on pasture.

Because cattle do not graze randomly on the pasture, the dung is not evenly distributed [23]. When the pasture is adequate, the cattle tend to avoid the area around the dung pat, resulting in plumes of grass around the pat. Larvae have adapted by migrating away from the pat, enhancing their chance of being ingested. When cattle are grazed intensively, they are forced to consume all of the available forage, increasing the numbers of larvae ingested.

Parasite dynamics in the host

When the infectious sheathed third-stage larvae are ingested, the worm development resumes. Exposure of the infectious larvae to the conditions of the rumen induces exsheathment of the larvae and signals parasite development [24,25]. The initial step in the infectious process is the shedding of the sheath remaining from the second-stage larvae, which occurs rapidly after the larvae are ingested. Studies in vitro show that within minutes after exposure to carbon dioxide or a mild hypochlorite solution, the larvae emerge from the second-stage sheath to resume development. Development from the now-parasitic third-stage larvae to reproductive adults varies in duration among the nematode species that infect ruminants.

Because *O ostertagi* is perhaps the most intensively studied species, it can be used to illustrate the dynamics of infection. Within 48 to 72 hours postinfection, the parasitic third-stage larvae are established in the gastric glands of the abomasum [26,27]. Between 96 and 120 hours postinfection, the larvae begin molting to the fourth-stage parasite. This stage is where arrestment occurs if development includes an arrestment phase. If the larvae do not exhibit an arrested phase, they will begin their final molt to the adult phase at 10 to 11 days postinfection [27]. At this point, some of the young adults may leave the gastric glands and establish residence in the gut lumen, but most parasites will remain in the glands and continue development. Beginning about 15 days postinfection, with a peak at about 17 days postinfection, the bulk of the new adult worms will tear their way out of the tissues, resulting in very characteristic clinical signs, including inappetence and a profuse, watery, and foul-smelling diarrhea. The adult worms will establish themselves in the lumen of the abomasum, mate, and then the females will begin laying eggs. In experimental *Ostertagia* infections, eggs begin to appear in the feces between 17 and 21 days postinfection, with peak production between 28 and approximately 40 days postinfection. At this time, egg production will rapidly decrease, reaching very low levels within approximately 8 to 9 weeks postinfection. Without treatment, eggs can appear sporadically in the feces for several months. Although the exact times of these developmental points are less well defined in other nematodes species, the pre-patent periods of the most common species are 3 to 4 weeks for *Cooperia* sp; 17 to 21 days for *Haemonchus contortus*; approximately 5 weeks for *Haemonchus placei*; 5 to 6 weeks for *Nematodirus helvetianus*; and 5 to 6 weeks for *Oesophagostomum radiatum*.

Once established in the gut lumen, the worms will actively feed. Some species, such as *H contortus,* are active blood feeders, whereas others, such as *Ostertagia*, ingest tissues and fluids from the mucosal surface, resulting in a denuding of the mucosa and, especially in the region near the pyloric sphincter, causing the surface of the mucosa to appear bloody and raw. For intestinal worms, profound changes in the macro- and microarchitecture of the gut are characteristic of nematode infections. In murine models, infection causes profound changes in the columnar epithelia lining the gut, reduces height and number of microvilli on the luminal surface of the lining epithelial cells, increases numbers of goblet cells in the mucosa, increases thickness and cell numbers in the muscularis layer, and causes influx of inflammatory cells into the submucosa [28]. Physiologically, the gut becomes hyperactive. Peristalsis increases in frequency and strength of contractions, neural components become more sensitive and therefore require weaker signals to react, and fluids are actively transported out of the tissues into the lumen. The overall result is an animal with a decreased appetite, decreased gut retention time, and a net fluid, electrolyte, and nutrient loss to the gut lumen.

Although little is known about the life span of the various nematode species, most parasite species can clearly persist for several months in their host. Several factors influence survival of the parasites. Factors that shorten their life span can include the immune status of the host and the intensity of acquisition of new parasites [29]. Animals with substantial previous exposure to the parasites and those grazing in areas of high parasite numbers will turnover individual parasites faster than naive or lightly exposed animals. In addition, previous exposure to the parasites can induce structural changes in worms from subsequent infection (ie, loss of the vulval flap in *Ostertagia* females), and definitely reduces egg output of worms arising from later infections.

Benefits of effective control: economic impact

Economics of gastrointestinal nematode infections in the United States

The United States cattle herd consists of approximately 100 million cattle, of which approximately 10 million are milk cows. These livestock resources are valued at approximately $100 billion [30]. Gastrointestinal (GI) nematode infections are ubiquitous and among the most costly diseases in the cattle industry. Conservative estimates show that GI nematode parasites cost the American cattle industry more than $2 billion per year in lost productivity and increased operating expenses. This estimate is based on the assumption that most cattle in the United States receive an average of slightly more than one treatment per year, resulting in annual expenditures for anthelmintics of almost $500 million, with losses in productivity accounting for the remaining costs. Although these losses are difficult to measure directly if looking at the voluminous literature concerning enhanced weight gains seen immediately after treatment, treated animals show an average weight gain of between 5 and 10 kg, whereas lactating animals increase production by 1 to 2 kg/d. This estimate does not include the costs of labor associated with increased animal handling. Whether producers involved in all aspects of the American cattle industry and attending veterinarians recognize the potential of GI nematodes to cause economic loss is unclear.

The latest Cow/Calf Health and Productivity Audit performed by the Animal and Plant Health Inspection Service of United States Department of Agriculture asked cow/calf producers about "diseases or conditions that may have a significant economic impact on their operation" [31]. The number one (53.1%) and number three (47.3%) answers were external and internal parasites, respectively. Open- and late-calving cows (47.4%) was the only other condition mentioned by at least 25% of the respondents. In addition, nearly three of four producers (72.8%) used a dewormer in the previous year, with no indication of regional differences in this health practice, making this clearly the most prevalent treatment or vaccination for disease in cattle. Similarly, nearly all feedlots (98.9% with less than 8000 animals; 100% with more than 8000 animals) use a parasiticide in their operation [32]. Finally, in the most recent U.S. National Animal Health Monitoring System (NAHMS) survey [33], 69% of dairies administered anthelmintics to their replacement dairy heifers, whereas 60.3% used anthelmintics on their lactating animals.

Economics of gastrointestinal nematode infections on the farm

The effects of parasites on groups of individual animals impact the bottom line for producers; parasites negatively affect the economics of raising cattle. The economic impact of parasitism is commonly measured by comparing production in parasitized cattle with production of those that had their parasite burdens removed with an anthelmintic. These controlled studies evaluate a wide variety of parameters, from weight gains in stockers and dairy replacement heifers to weaning weights in cow/calf and milk production in dairy and beef cattle.

A four-site study of stocker cattle by Ballweber and colleagues [34] showed that over 140 days, the treatment groups experienced differences in weight gains of 0.152 to 0.272 kg/d compared with the control groups. Williams and colleagues [35] reported similar findings in cattle treated with doramectin, eprinomectin, ivermectin, or moxidectin compared with untreated controls, showing an average daily gain (ADG) advantage over the control ranging from 0.11 to 0.23 kg/d. Stromberg and colleagues [36] observed similar weaning weight advantages in cow/calf operations. The calves of treated dams were found to out-gain the control calves by 19.3 and 13.2 kg in each of two successive years ($P < .0001$) in Minnesota. After adjusting for birthweight and birth date, treated calves showed an ADG of 0.13 kg more than the controls. This study also observed a significant increase in reproductive performance of the cows ($P = .0357$). The pregnancy rate averaged across the 2 years was 94% for the treated cows compared with 82% for the control animals. A similar study in Georgia found a weaning weight advantage of 0.04 kg ADG over the controls. They also noted an improvement in pregnancy rates of the parasite-free cows compared with controls (98% vs. 75%) [37].

Although the economic value of improved reproductive performance is difficult to calculate, the differences in ADG can be used to calculate a return on investment for a producer when the advantage of the ADG for parasite-free calves, the value of kilograms of calf-weight sold, the number of days on pasture (study), the cost of the product, and an appropriate cattle handling charge are known. These production advantages when parasites are removed result in increased profit to the producer. They also result in significantly reduced parasite egg shedding and pasture contamination.

Dairy replacement heifers, like grazing beef cattle, grow better when they are parasite-free. Elsner and colleagues [38], for example, reported a gain advantage of 16 kg over 143 days. Parasite-free cattle may also benefit dairy operations by increasing milk production, although data seem to be more variable. A review of 87 studies that evaluated the impact of anthelmintic treatment and parasite removal on milk production found that 80% of the studies showed a significant increase in milk production [39], with a median increase of 0.63 kg/d. Ploeger and colleagues [40] observed that cows that were treated to remove parasites produced 132.9 kg milk per cow per lactation more than their parasitized cohorts. A study by Gibb and colleagues [41] found that parasite removal yielded an increase in solids of 1.68 kg/d corrected milk ($P = .026$). Only anthelmintics that are approved for use in lactating dairy animals must be used. Milk production in beef cattle also seems to be increased, and may partially explain calf growth in the early part of the grazing season. A significant ($P < .05$) increase in milk production occurred in beef cows after anthelmintic treatment. Treated cows produced an average of 3.49 kg milk per suckling versus 2.76 kg per suckling for the untreated cows using the weigh–suckle–weigh method [42].

Effects of nematodes on the host

The interaction of cattle and their GI nematode parasites can result in several physiologic responses that negatively impact animal production and well-being. These responses arise from the direct destructive effect of the parasites on host tissues, and more indirect responses, such as a potential suppression of immune responses unrelated to parasite antigens or immunopathology.

Perhaps the single most economically important direct physiologic response is a loss of appetite by the infected host. Infected animals, whether on pasture or in a confined feeding operation, show a reduced feed intake compared with uninfected animals. This loss of appetite may be caused by several factors, including abdominal pain, the secretion of inflammatory chemokines by immunocompetent cells, or the stimulation of regulatory hormones, such as gastrin, by the infected gut [43].

In addition to a decreased nutrient intake, the normal digestive process is also affected. Parasites have several direct effects on gut tissues, of which the best characterized is perhaps destruction of the gastric glands by larval *Ostertagia*. As the larvae mature from the infective third stage to the young adult within the gastric glands, the gland itself is destroyed and becomes nonfunctional. This destruction includes loss of secretory cells and alterations of the epithelium, including a loss of integrity of the cell junctional complexes leading to leakage of pepsinogen into the general circulation [44]. These changes cause interference in the host's protein digestion. As the young adults exit the destroyed glands, they create massive damage. Although the infective larvae are small and can enter the gland with no tissue damage, the young adults leave the glands by tearing through the tissues, leaving a raw and bloody mucosal surface. In the intestine, parasites such as *Cooperia* may induce profound tissue changes that cause fluid, electrolyte, and protein losses [45]. The combination of anorexia, disruption of normal digestion, and loss of tissue fluids results in an extremely inefficient production animal [46].

In addition to the direct destructive effects of the parasites, infections with GI nematodes can markedly interfere with the host immune system and may render the animal less able to respond immunologically to other infectious agents or vaccinations. This decreased immunocompetence may be caused by multiple pathways. Evidence exists that a hyperstimulation (ie, polyclonal activation of certain cell types) may divert the immune response of cattle infected with GI nematodes [47]. Additionally, GI nematodes are extraordinarily effective stimulators of immune responses mediated by T-helper type 2 (Th2) lymphocytes [45]. However, because Th2 cytokines are counter-regulatory for immune responses mediated by T-helper type 1 (Th1) lymphocytes, important responses, such as certain antiviral responses, may be impaired [45]. Finally, GI nematodes can produce and release substances that are potent immunomodulators [48,49] that can directly interfere with immunocompetent cells near the site of infection.

Therefore, GI nematodes can exert several effects on cattle that can significantly impair the overall health and well-being of the host, including direct effects on the digestion and absorption of needed nutrients, and indirect effects on the host immune system that may cause a decreased ability to respond to other infectious agents or decreased productivity from an exaggerated stimulation of the gut immune system.

Chemical control

Deworming programs

Therapeutic or *curative deworming* occurs when cattle are treated with an anthelmintic in response to increased egg counts or when cattle are visibly being impacted by parasites. This practice may be recommended by a veterinarian or consultant or may be performed when the producer observes that the animals are not growing as expected or have a rough hair coat or bottle jaw, in which case individual animals or the entire herd are dewormed with an anthelmintic. Deworming treatments may be repeated at varying intervals, and although dosing may become more frequent, treatments can still be provided with little if any plan.

Preventative deworming (multidosing) is three or more treatments at regular intervals of 6 weeks or less [50], and may be as frequent as 2-week intervals for up to 2 to 3 months. An increased number of treatments may lead to suppressive deworming, with the goal of keeping the parasites and pasture burden at a minimal level [51]. The benefits of multidosing include increased weight gains and, in some cases, simply keeping the animals alive. However, in addition to being expensive, this method has the potential for selecting for resistance to the compound involved [52].

Suppressive therapy is multidosing that prevents adult parasite populations from developing to maturity and contaminating the pasture. For example, animals in Australia were treated with an anthelmintic to effectively suppress egg shedding for an entire grazing season [111]. A similar effect may also be achieved with a sustained release product.

Recent developments include new forms of continuous release methodologies. One of the first was the *sustained release* (SR) morantel bolus, which provided continuous dosing over an extended period. Craig and colleagues [53] observed that the bolus provided parasite control and significant weight gain advantages compared with the parasitized calves during the 168-day study period. Years later, an ivermectin SR bolus was developed that was reported to reduce parasite egg shedding for 230 days and provide significant weight gains compared with control groups [54]. More recently, *long-acting injectable* products are being developed, such as the moxidectin product described by Ranjan and colleagues [55] that reduced infection by more than 98% when hosts were challenged with infective larvae 150 days after administration of the anthelmintic. Subsequent field studies showed persistent activity against several species of cattle nematodes [56]. A preliminary report of another long-acting injectable product was reported using eprinomectin [57].

Management practices alone can reduce parasite burdens by creating safe pastures, usually through resting the pasture for various periods. Safe pastures are those that have a lowered risk for infection because reduced numbers of infective larvae are present on the herbage. This lowered risk may be accomplished by moving cattle to new pastures after periods of peak contamination and allowing the pasture to lie fallow for sufficient time to reduce parasite numbers. This practice allows the larvae to die off during periods when the pasture is not grazed [58,59], taking advantage of the weather to reduce larval numbers. Experts have assumed that few larvae survive the harsh summers in the south [13] or the harsh winters in the north [60]. However, recoveries from tracer calves showed that although the population of pasture larvae decreased from July to the following April, some were still available after a harsh Minnesota winter [19]. Likewise, larvae were shown to survive the midsummer heat in Southern California [61], but few survived the harsh summers in Louisiana [13]. Adverse weather has a negative impact on larval numbers and provides some degree of parasite control by reducing larval numbers and thus the infection pressure.

The practice of moving cattle to the aftermath of harvested crops such as wheat, corn, soybeans, or cotton has been shown to offer safe pasture [62]. These pastures have been tilled, planted, and harvested since they were last grazed. Few studies have evaluated the interaction of the herbage species and larval dynamics.

The next logical step in controlling ruminant helminths seems to be to combine pasture management with a deworming program. The dose and move (Weybridge) system, in which cattle are treated and moved to a clean safe pasture [62], was one of the first in the literature. Investigators in Australian and New Zealand have based control programs on reducing pasture contamination using antiparasitic compounds during what would have been peak parasite egg shedding [58,63]. Similar programs have been evaluated in North America [19,64,65]. The integrative approach by Williams and colleagues [51] combined the strategic use of an anthelmintic and grazing management with a consideration of the dynamics of the pasture and the larvae that live there. These programs, known as *strategic deworming*, use anthelmintics strategically to keep pasture burdens low and thus reduce the infection pressure on the host.

Anthelmintics are often used inappropriately. Products are often used suppressively to keep animals parasite-free. If the same product is used repeatedly, a resistant population of worms may be created. Overdosing and underdosing are also issues, which may be performed consciously with the idea that more is better or that a lesser dose of the product will still work effectively. Dosing based on estimated cattle weights rather than known weights often results in underestimating the weight and therefore underdosing the animals. Producers, by necessity, are very cost-conscious and often assume they can save money by underdosing (delivering less then the recommended dose), often resulting in failure to remove the dose-limiting parasites and exposing all worms to a subtherapeutic dose. Other producers assume that if *x* dose is recommended, then twice that dose will be even better. However, this method causes drug to be wasted (losing money), which will directly impact the bottom line (return on investment). Treating cattle when only a few parasites are present will also have little impact on pasture contamination and again may be considered a wasted treatment.

Resistance to anthelmintics and recommendations

The discovery of endectocides has profoundly influenced livestock production in the United States. Because of their large margin of safety, high efficacy, and broad range of activity, including both endo- and ectoparasites, they have influenced the manner and frequency of anthelmintic use and livestock-raising practices. The advent of the avermectins has coincided with the development of strategic treatment regimens that have the goal of achieving optimal animal productivity. This goal is accomplished through reducing parasite transmission by clearing pastures of infectious larvae. Combining highly efficacious and broad-range drugs with treatment programs that apply these drugs in a manner that maximizes reductions in parasite populations has led to several alterations in production practices, including higher stocking rates and reduced use of alternate control practices.

Although these programs have been profitable for many cattle raisers in the United States, concern exists that programs relying strictly on drug administration without regard for good pasture parasite management will lead to the selection of drug resistance in the nematode populations. This selection has been well documented in small ruminant species where GI nematodes resistant to all classes of anthelmintics, including the avermectins [66]. Because well-documented reports of drug resistance in cattle nematodes are scarce, some experts have postulated that because the immune system of cattle seems to handle GI nematode infections better than sheep and goats, resistance to the drugs in cattle parasites was unlikely caused by a lesser selective pressure from a lower drug usage [67]. Although this idea has been broadly held, anecdotal reports of lowered drug efficacy have increased and well-documented reports exist of drug resistance to the benzimidazoles in *Cooperia* spp in New Zealand [68,69], to ivermectin in *Cooperia* spp in Great Britain [70], and to both macrocyclic lactones and benzimidazoles in *Haemonchus* spp and the macrocyclic lactones in *Cooperia* spp in Argentina [71].

Until recently, none of these parasites has been seen in North America. Recent reports conclusively identified cattle nematodes showing resistance to all the commonly used avermectins and moxidectin in *Cooperia* spp and *Haemonchus* spp, and to the benzimidazoles in *H contortus* in cattle (Gasbarre and colleagues, submitted for publication). Increasing reports of apparently less-than-expected results on anthelmintic treatment coincide with this study. No conclusive evidence currently defines the level or extent of anthelmintic resistance in cattle nematodes in North America, but if anthelmintic resistance in cattle mimics the appearance of anthelmintic resistance in small ruminants, the problem would expand both geographically and in severity.

Current nematode control in cattle is primarily based on the use of either an avermectin or moxidectin, or a benzimidazole. Two older classes of anthelmintics are still available, but their use is uncommon. The available compounds from these older classes are levamisole and morantel tartrate. Because these drugs are seldom used today, the earlier studies tested levamisole on avermectin- and benzimidazole-resistant parasites, showing it to be efficacious. Although this treatment provides an option for producers in locations where these parasite forms are found, the abomasa of the group treated with levamisole hydrochloride contained *O ostertagi*, indicating that complete reliance on this drug should be undertaken carefully. Because levamisole is generally believed to be ineffective against larval *Ostertagia*, use of this drug alone might not adequately control *Ostertagia* numbers on pasture. Given the higher pathogenicity of *Ostertagia* compared with *Haemonchus* or *Cooperia* in cattle, reliance on this drug alone could lead to suboptimal control programs. In contrast, the combined use of levamisole and an avermectin seemed to be the most efficacious treatment in these studies.

Given the uncertainties surrounding the extent of anthelmintic resistance in cattle and the limited treatment options available, using complimentary classes of drug is recommended when producers are not satisfied with the treatment response. The combination of an avermectin or milbemycin with a benzimidazole or levamisole would be an effective cocktail with high efficacy against all important parasite species, and should also be effective against drug-resistant forms. A feedlot is another situation where these combinations might be appropriate, because all parasites must be removed to ensure maximal productivity and enhanced response to vaccination programs. However, because heavy indiscriminate anthelmintic use only hastens the appearance and spread of drug resistance in parasite populations, this treatment should be reserved for when treatment with a single class of drug seems ineffective, or in a feedlot situation. Because different modes of action are currently limited, and bringing a new drug to market requires extreme expense and time, unnecessary overapplication of the drugs could lead to severe problems for the American cattle industry.

Alternatives to chemical control

Immunity

Most cattle with sufficient previous exposure to GI nematodes can effectively limit the number of eggs released to pasture. Supporting evidence includes the observation that as cattle age, the EPG values for individuals decrease. Therefore, the mean EPG value for a cohort of calves is higher than that for a cohort of yearlings, which is higher than that for a cohort of cows all grazing the same pastures. Similarly, the same cohort of animals sampled as they age will show decreased mean EPG values when managed on the same pastures under similar management programs each succeeding year. These reductions in the number of parasite eggs released in the feces result from several different types of immune responses, ranging from those that alter parasite morphology or physiology to those that protect the host from reinfection, presumably through killing the developing worms or excluding the invasive third-stage larvae. These responses can usually be seen after animals have been on pasture for several months. Obviously, the ideal responses are those that reduce parasite numbers in the host without inducing immunopathology or interfering with animal productivity. Some GI nematode species, such as certain *Cooperia* and *Haemonchus* spp, seem to readily induce immune responses that significantly reduce the number of worms that become established in the grazing cattle.

One glaring exception is *O ostertagi*. Cattle remain susceptible to infection by this parasite for many months, and immunity that actually reduces the number of newly acquired larvae that develop is usually not evident after prolonged exposure [72] and may not be seen until the animals are older than 2 years. Similarly, as many as five repeated drug-attenuated infections are required to achieve a significant reduction (approximately 72%) in mean worm counts compared with the primary infected groups [73]. This prolonged susceptibility to reinfection is a major reason that *O ostertagi* remains the most economically important GI nematode in the United States. Although the animals remain susceptible to reinfection for a prolonged period, the immune system causes a stunting in the newly acquired worms, and the female worms produce significantly fewer eggs than those in a primary infection, resulting in reduced parasite transmission or enhanced herd immunity.

The reasons for this delayed onset of protective immunity directed against *O ostertagi* are unclear. On infection, *O ostertagi* can elicit profound changes in the host immune systems, including a rapid and enormous expansion of lymphocytes and lymphoid cells, increased expression of interleukin (IL)-4, and extensive changes in the abomasal tissue and its draining lymph nodes [47,74–76]. Studies using rodent–nematode models strongly suggest that immunity to GI nematode infections is a strong inducer of a stereotypic immune response mediated by Th2 lymphocytes. The rodent–nematode and the cattle–*Ostertagia* systems seem to have several differences. *Ostertagia* infection does not seem to induce a typical Th2 response in cattle. A primary infection induces IL-4 and interferon gamma (IFN-γ), which is a Th1 cytokine, in the abomasal lymph node [75]. Additionally, although IL-4 is directly involved in protective immunity in rodents, it may not be associated with the protective mechanism against *O ostertagi* in cattle [73]. The type of response elicited may be dose-dependent, in that trickle infections seem to induce a response more characteristic of a Th2 paradigm [77]. Finally, although rapid expulsion of resident adult parasites is a major protective mechanism against intestinal nematodes in mice, no evidence of rapid expulsion of the parasite has been documented in the cattle–*Ostertagia* system.

Potential mechanisms have been proposed for this unique weak protective immunity induced by *Ostertagia* [78], among which immunosuppression has been the most thoroughly investigated. *Ostertagia* may have developed means to actively suppress or evade the host immune system. *Ostertagia* infection can exhibit nonspecific and antigen-specific suppressive effects on the host immune response. Suppressive molecules exist in extracts of third-stage and fourth-stage larvae [48,49]. The parasite can depress T-cell responses while B-cell responses remain normal [79,80]. Concurrent with this immunosuppression are increases in the percentage of B cells and γδ T cells at the sites of infection (abomasal mucosa and lymph nodes) and a decrease in αβ T cells [74]. Polyclonal B-cell activation may also be involved because these responses are common in parasitic diseases [47].

Future development of immunologic tools, such as vaccines or immunomodulators, to protect cattle from infection may be feasible for certain nematode parasites [81]. The value of this approach is currently limited by the ability of nematodes such as *Ostertagia* to evade host-immune responses [78]. As these evasive mechanisms are better understood, procedures to ablate or lessen these immunoregulatory activities can be devised. A continuing problem with immunotherapy (ie, vaccines or immunomodulators) will be the requirement that treatment confer protection against all important parasite species in a given locality while fitting within producer guidelines regarding cost and labor required.

Genetics of gastrointestinal nematode infections

As animals age, the number of eggs they release in their feces decreases. An additional factor affecting parasite numbers and egg shedding by cattle is the genetic makeup of the animal. Firstly, the sex of the animal influences EPG values, with bulls having higher EPG values than cows [82,83]. Perhaps most importantly, EPG values are not normally distributed within a cattle herd. Instead, the values follow a distribution termed an *overdispered distribution* [84–87]. This overdispered distribution is characterized by the value of the standard error of the mean exceeding the value of the mean. In this distribution, most individuals have low fecal EPG values, and a small percentage of animals are responsible for most of the eggs released on the pastures, resulting in animals that can be classified as parasite susceptible or "nonresponders." These animals are usually estimated to constitute between 15% and 25% of the total population [86,88]. One result of the overdispersion of parasites in a cattle herd is the need to use proper sampling techniques if trying to estimate the true mean EPG value for a group of animals. If the susceptible or high EPG animals are assumed to constitute approximately 15% to 25% of a particular age group (eg, calves, yearlings), then the subset sampled must contain one or more of these animals that will have a disproportionally large effect on the herd mean. To ensure that the high-EPG animals are included, between 17 and 20 random samples must be collected from any group of cattle regardless of the total number of animals [89]. This recommendation assumes that the samples are collected randomly, and that an individual animal is not sampled more than once. If the group has less than 17 animals, then all members of the group should be sampled.

The observation that fecal egg counts are not normally distributed within cattle populations raised the possibility that host genetics might influence parasite infection levels in cattle. A series of experiments showed that the EPG of pastured cattle was influenced by host genetics [90], and that the heritability of this trait was approximately 0.30 [82], indicating that the trait is moderately heritable (with approximately the same heritability as milk production in cattle). Additionally, other studies indicated that certain bulls had 20 times greater odds of producing susceptible (high-EPG) calves than other bulls [91].

Further studies using animals selected for enhanced resistance or extreme susceptibility to nematode infections showed several important characteristics. First, cattle can be separated into three phenotypes: (1) one that never shows high EPG values when placed on infected pastures, (2) one that shows increased EPG values through the first 2 to 3 months after exposure to infected pastures, and then decreased EPG values to a level seen in innately resistant cattle, and (3) one that maintains high EPG levels throughout their residence on infected pastures. Secondly, the best indicator of level of *Cooperia* infection was the EPG value ($r = 0.6$), whereas *Ostertagia* was best measured by serum pepsinogen levels ($r = 0.7$), weight gain ($r = -0.5$), and measures of anemia ($r = 0.5$). Other phenotypic measures were poor predictors of parasite numbers [92]. These relationships agree with reports of similar parasite–host systems [93,94]. In contrast, studies in tropical areas have indicated significant correlations between fecal EPG values and total worm numbers [95]. This difference is probably because of the reduced presence of *Ostertagia* in tropical environments.

Current efforts are directed toward using modern methods in genomic analysis to identify the natural genetic variation that underlies resistance and susceptibility to GI nematodes, and the characterization of molecular markers for this trait. Accurate knowledge of genes controlling resistance will offer producers alternatives for disease control. For nonorganic producers, susceptible animals can be targeted for drug administration. This approach reduces the cost of anthelmintics used and the likelihood of drug resistance. A second option is to target susceptible animals for immunotherapy involving vaccines or immunomodulation once the precise immunologic pathways are elucidated. A final option is selection to remove susceptible animals from the herd; producers at high risk for parasite-induced production losses, such as organic producers or those in geographic areas with high rates of transmission, would benefit most from this strategy. In contrast, producers in areas or using management systems where the impact of the parasites is less severe could choose to select against susceptibility within the broader breeding goals of their programs.

Novel methods for controlling helminths

Efforts to identify novel methods for reducing helminth numbers and satisfying the needs of organic and sustainable producers are gaining popularity. This effort is driven by the nonchemical needs of the organic producers and the need to find alternative means of controlling worms because of increasing resistance to many of the currently used anthelmintics. These novel methods include using natural compounds, modulating the host immune response, and using host insusceptibility to understand more of the host's genetics [96].

Natural compounds

The predaceous microfungi, such as *Duddingtonia flagrans*, have been studied for their ability to reduce or restrict nematode parasitism. These fungi prey on the pasture larvae as a food source and thus reduce the overall pasture larval population. The advantages of these fungi, identified by Waller and Thamsborg [97], are that they survive passage through the bovine GI tract and grow rapidly in fresh dung. Therefore, the fungus can break the life cycle by capturing the developing larval stages before they migrate out onto the pasture to infect animals. Although this area of parasite control is still in development, numerous studies have shown the potential of this biologic control method [98,99]. These investigators found that *D flagrans* significantly reduced the number of free-living lungworm and GI larvae. Although studies by Waller and colleagues [100] showed that this concept works under field conditions, other studies suggested little if any significant impact in the field [101].

Evidence exists that plant materials, such as tannins (plant polyphenols), have some antiparasitic effect on ruminant helminths. Waller and Thamsborg [97] referred to these materials as *plant nutraceuticals*. Most studies have been conducted in sheep and goats, and they have shown better efficacy against the intestinal worms than against those in the abomasum [102]. Field studies of animals that grazed on tannin-rich pastures showed improved performance and reduced parasitism compared with those raised on tannin-free pastures. Chicory (*Cichorium intybus*), a compound that was used for parasite control before modern anthelmintics were developed, has recently shown efficacy against abomasal nematodes in sheep [103]. Although this area is still being actively investigated and is still in its infancy, it is promising as a potential aid in reducing parasite numbers.

Plant cysteine proteinases were also reported to have activity against some helminths. These proteolytic enzymes are obtained from the fruits and latex of plants such as papaya, fig, and pineapple. They have low toxicity and their enzymatic activity has been reported to digest away the nematode cuticle [104]. Further investigation is needed to confirm any practical benefit of this traditional helminth control. Tagboto and Townson [105] reviewed the antiparasitic properties of plants and other natural products.

Copper oxide wire particles have been known for their antiparasitic activity since the 1960s. These particles are currently being reevaluated for their ability to prevent the establishment of abomasal worms and for their inhibitory effect on worm fecundity in sheep [106,107]. The greatest effect seems to be in *H contortus*. Studies conducted in Sweden found little if any benefit to using the copper wire bolus in sheep [108]. One of the few studies evaluating copper wire particles in cattle also found they had limited activity against GI worms [109].

Efforts to identify natural compounds that will actually reduce helminth numbers and satisfy the organic producers have also increased. An older compound that is often identified by producers is diatomaceous earth. Numerous anecdotal accounts exist of its efficacy, although little actual evidence of efficacy. Fernandez and colleagues [110] found little if any difference between fecal egg counts for diatomaceous earth–treated cattle and untreated controls.

Summary

Nematode infections in ruminants can be managed with numerous control strategies. By necessity, many current methods of control are reactionary as the parasites acquire resistance to anthelmintics. However, as new classes of compounds with new modes of action become available, these chemistries must be used in a way that maximizes efficacy but also prolongs the life of the compounds. This practice should include managing the herd genetics and immune responses against the parasites in combination with the judicious and timely use of anthelmintics. Future programs may also control helminths with combined approaches, such as pasture larval control (using fungi), providing forages with antiparasite activity, and managing host genetics and immunity. These programs must be integrated so they do not rely on any single method, because the parasites have an astounding ability to evolve mechanisms to elude the current therapy. A hallmark of any parasite–host system is the extraordinary ability of the parasites to adapt to new challenges. Continued cost-effective parasite management must also show a level of high adaptability.

References

[1] Stromberg BE. Environmental factors influencing transmission. Vet Parasitol 1997;72:247–64.

[2] Ciordia H, Bizzell WE. The effects of various constant temperatures on the development of free living-stages of some nematode parasites of cattle. J Parasitol 1963;49:60–3.

[3] Enigk K, Dey-Harza A. In: Levine ND, editor. Chapter 6. Trichostrongyles. Nematode parasites of domestic animals and man. Minneapolis (MN): Burgess; 1980. p. 163.

[4] Ciordia H, Bizzell WE, Porter DA, et al. The effect of culture temperature and age on the infectivity of the larvae of *Trichostrongylus axei* and *T. colubriformis* in rabbits and guinea pigs. J Parasitol 1966;52:866–70.

[5] Levine ND. Weather, climate and the bionomics of ruminant nematode larvae. Adv Vet Sci Comp Med 1963;19:215–61.

[6] Goldberg A. Development and survival on pasture of gastrointestinal nematode parasites of cattle. J Parasitol 1968;54:856–62.

[7] Williams JC, Mayhew RL. Survival of infective larvae of the cattle nematodes, *Cooperia punctata*, *Trichostrongylus axei*, and *Oesophagostomum radiatum*. Am J Vet Res 1967;28:629–40.

[8] Lancaster MD, Hong C. Observations on the pattern of nematode availability on pasture grazed annually by cattle, 1959–1985. Vet Rec 1987;120:502–3.
[9] Bryan RP, Kerr JD. Factors affecting the survival and migration of the free-living stages of gastrointestinal nematode parasites of cattle in central Queensland. Vet Parasitol 1989;30: 315–26.
[10] Krecek RC, Murrell KD, Douglas LW. Effects of microclimate variables on the availability and movement of third-stage larvae of *Ostertagia ostertagi* on herbage. Onderstepoort J Vet Res 1990;57:133–5.
[11] Tarshis IB. A preliminary study of the lateral migration by infective larvae of some cattle nematodes on experimentally contaminated forage plots. Proc Helm Soc Wash 1958;25: 99–106.
[12] Levine ND, Todd KS, Boatman PA. Development and survival of *Haemonchus contortus* on pasture. Am J Vet Res 1974;35:1413–22.
[13] Williams JC, Bilkovich FR. Distribution of *Ostertagia ostertagi* infective larvae on pasture herbage. Am J Vet Res 1973;34:1337–44.
[14] Crofton HD. The ecology of immature phases of trichostrongyle nematodes. Parasitol 1948;39:17–25.
[15] Silangwa SM, Todd AC. Vertical migration of trichostrongyle larvae in grasses. J Parasitol 1964;50:278–85.
[16] Krecek RC, Murrell KD. Observations on the ability of larval *Ostertagia ostertagi* to migrate through pasture soil. Proc Helminthol Soc Wash 1988;55:24–7.
[17] Grønvold J, Høgh-Schmidt K. Factors influencing rain splash dispersal of infective larvae of Ostertagia ostertagi (Trichostrongylidae) from cow pats to the surroundings. Vet Parasitol 1989;31:57–70.
[18] Grønvold J. Rain splash dispersal of third-stage larvae of *Cooperia* spp. (Trichostrongylidae). J Parasitol 1984;70:924–6.
[19] Stromberg BE, Schlotthauer JC, Haggard DL, et al. The epizootiology of helminth parasitism in a Minnesota beef cow/calf herd. Am J Vet Res 1991;52:1712–6.
[20] Fincher GT. Dung beetles as biological control agents for gastrointestinal parasites of livestock. J Parasitol 1973;59:396–9.
[21] Fincher GT. Effects of dung beetle activity on the number of nematode parasites acquired by grazing cattle. J Parasitol 1975;61:759–62.
[22] Bergstrom RC, Maki LR, Werner BA. Small dung beetles as biological control agents: laboratory studies of beetle action on trichostrongylid eggs in sheep and cattle feces. Proc Helm Soc Wash 1976;43:171–4.
[23] Bryan RP, Kerr JD. The grazing behavior of cattle in relation to the sampling of infective nematode larvae on pasture. Vet Parasitol 1988;30:73–82.
[24] Rodgers WP, Somerville RI. The infective process and its relation to the development of early parasitic stages of nematodes. Adv Parasitol 1968;6:327–48.
[25] Somerville RI, Rodgers WP. The nature and action of host signals. Adv Parasitol 1987;26: 239–93.
[26] Gasbarre LC. Recovery of larval *Ostertagia ostertagi* from the abomasa of experimentally inoculated calves by prolonged saline incubation. Proc Helminthol Soc Wash 1987;54: 160–1.
[27] Canals A, Gasbarre LC. Procedure for the recovery of excretory-secretory products of from molting fourth-stage larvae of *Ostertagia ostertagi*. Proc Helm Soc Wash 1989;56: 201–3.
[28] Castro GA. Physiology of the gastrointestinal tract in the parasitized host. In: Johnson LR, editor. Physiology of the gastrointestinal tract. New York: Raven Press; 1981. p. 1381–406.
[29] Michel JF. Some observations on the worm burdens of calves infected daily with Ostertagia ostertagi. Parasitology 1969;59:575–95.
[30] Economic Research Service, USDA. Available at: http://www.ers.usda.gov/. Accessed July 9, 2006.

[31] National Animal Health Monitoring System, USDA. Beef '97: Part III: reference of 1997 beef cow-calf production management and disease control. Fort Collins (CO): US Dept. of Agriculture, APHIS; 1998.
[32] National Animal Health Monitoring System, USDA. Part III. health management and biosecurity on U.S feedlots, 1999. Fort Collins (CO): US Dept. of Agriculture, APHIS; 2000.
[33] National Animal Health Monitoring System, USDA. Dairy 2002: Part II: changes in the United States dairy industry, 1991–2002. Fort Collins (CO): US Dept. of Agriculture, APHIS; 2002.
[34] Ballweber LR, Smith LL, Stuedemann JA, et al. The effectiveness of a single treatment with doramectin or ivermectin in the control of gastrointestinal nematodes in grazing yearling stocker cattle. Vet Parasitol 1997;72:53–68.
[35] Williams JC, Loyacano AF, DeRosa A, et al. A comparison of persistent anthelmintic efficacy of topical formulations of doramectin, ivermectin, eprinomectin and moxidectin against naturally acquired nematode infections of beef calves. Vet Parasitol 1999;85: 277–88.
[36] Stromberg BE, Vatthauer RJ, Schlotthauer JC, et al. Production responses following strategic parasite control in a beef cow/calf herd. Vet Parasitol 1997;68:315–22.
[37] Stuedeman JA, Ciordia H, Myers GH, et al. Effect of a single strategically timed dose of fenbendazole on cow and calf performance. Vet Parasitol 1989;34:77–86.
[38] Elsener J, Villeneuve A, DesCoteaux L. Evaluation of a strategic deworming program in dairy heifers in Quebec based on the use of moxidectin, an endectocide with a long persistency. Can Vet J 2001;42:38–44.
[39] Gross SJ, Ryan WG, Ploeger HW. Anthelmintic treatment of dairy cows and its effect on milk production. Vet Rec 1999;144:581–7.
[40] Ploeger HW, Kloosterman A, Bargeman G, et al. Milk yield increase after anthelmintic treatment of dairy cattle related to some parameters estimating helminth infection. Vet Parasitol 1990;35:103–16.
[41] Gibb MJ, Huckle CA, Forbes AB. Effects of sequential treatments with eprinomectin on performance and grazing behavior in dairy cattle under daily-paddock stocking management. Vet Parasitol 2005;133:79–90.
[42] Stromberg BE, Corwin RM. Epizootiology of *Ostertagia ostertagi* in cow-calf production systems in the American Midwest. Vet Parasitol 1993;46:297–302.
[43] Fox MT, Carroll AP, Hughes SA, et al. Gastrin and gastrin-related responses to infection with *Ostertagia ostertagi* in the calf. Res Vet Sci 1993;54:384–91.
[44] Murray M. Structural changes in bovine ostertagiasis associated with increased permeability of the bowel wall to macromoleclues. Gastroenterol 1969;56:763–72.
[45] Finkelman FD, Shea-Donohue T, Morris SC, et al. Interleukin-4- and interleukin-13-mediated host protection against intestinal nematode parasites. Immunol Rev 2004;201: 139–55.
[46] Simpson HV. Pathophysiology of abomasal parasitism: Is the host or parasite responsible. Vet J 2000;160:177–91.
[47] Gasbarre LC. Limiting dilution analyses for the quantification of cellular immune responses in bovine ostertagiasis. Vet Parasitol 1986;20:133–47.
[48] Cross DA, Klesius PH. Soluble extracts from larval *Ostertagia* ostertagi modulating immune function. Int J Parasitol 1989;1(1):57–61.
[49] Gomez-Munoz MT, Canals-Caballero A, Almeria S, et al. Inhibition of bovine T lymphocyte responses by extracts of the stomach worm Ostertagia ostertagi. Vet Parasitol 2004; 120(3):199–214.
[50] Morley FHW, Donald AD. Farm management and systems of helminth control. Vet Parasitol 1980;6:105–34.
[51] Williams JC, Corwin RM, Craig TM, et al. Control strategies for nematodiasis in cattle. Vet Clin North Am Food Anim Pract 1986;2:247–60.

[52] Gasbarre LC, Smith LL, Pillit PA. Identification of cattle nematode parasites resistant to multiple classes of anthelmintics in a commercial cattle population in the US [abstract 46]. In: Proc Am Assoc Vet Parasitol 50th Annual Meeting 2005:57. Abstract.
[53] Craig TM, Field RW, Rupp GP. Use of the sustained-release morantel bolus in stocker calves in southern United States. Am J Vet Res 1988;49(10):1729–32.
[54] Ballweber LR, Brown J, Hawkins JA, et al. Comparison of ivermectin SR bolus, benzimidazole anthelmintics, and topical fenthion on productivity of stocker cattle from grazing through feedlot. Vet Therap 2000;1(3):192–8.
[55] Ranjan S, Szewczyk E, Search R, et al. Evaluation of the period of protection of 10% moxidectin cattle long-acting against *D. viviparus, H. placei, T. axei* and *O. radiatum* infection in cattle [abstract 167]. In: Proceedings of the XIX International Conference of the WAAVP 2003:184. Abstract.
[56] Yazwinski TA, Williams JC, Smith LL, et al. Dose determination of the persistent activity of moxidectin long-acting injectable formulations against various nematode species in cattle. Vet Parasitol 2006;137:273–85.
[57] Marley SE, Kunkle B, Holste JE, et al. Persistent 120-day efficacy and dose confirmation of eprinomectin in a long-acting injection (EpLAI) against adult and developing GI and/or pulmonary nematodes in cattle [abstract 43]. In: Proc Am Assoc Vet Parasitol 50th Annual Meeting 2005:55. Abstract.
[58] Brundson RV. Principles of helminth control. Vet Parasitol 1980;6:185–215.
[59] Donald A. Some recent advances in the epidemiology and control of helminth infection in sheep. Proc Aust Soc Anim Prod 1974;10:148–55.
[60] Gibbs HC. Persistence on pasture of infective larvae of nematodes parasitizing Maine dairy cattle. Am J Vet Res 1980;51:1694–5.
[61] Baker NF, Fisk RA. Seasonal occurrence of infective nematode larvae in California Sierra foothills grazed by cattle. Am J Vet Res 1986;47:1680–5.
[62] Michel JF. The epidemiology and control of some nematode infections in grazing animals Adv Parasitol 1976;14:355–97.
[63] Anderson N. The epidemiology and control of bovine ostertagiasis in a winter rainfall region of southeastern Australia. In: Ostertagia Symposium 80. Australia: Roseworthy Agricultural College, Roseworthy South Australia; 1980. p. 63–9.
[64] Myers GH, Todd AC. Increased weight gains of Wisconsin dairy heifers following systematic deworming with fenbendazole. Am J Vet Res 1980;41:1886–9.
[65] Hawkins JA, Evans RR, Newby TJ, et al. Field efficacy of morantel sustained release bolus for control of gastrointestinal nematodes in yearling steers. Vet Parasitol 1985;17: 229–38.
[66] Waller PJ. Anthelmintic resistance. Vet Parasitol 1997;72:391–412.
[67] Waller PJ. The development of anthelmintic resistance in ruminant livestock. Acta Trop 1994;56:233–43.
[68] Vermunt JJ, West DM, Pomroy WE. Multiple resistance to ivermectin and oxfendazole in *Cooperia* species of cattle in New Zealand. Vet Rec 1995;137:43–5.
[69] Hosking BC, Watson TG, Leathwick DM. Multigeneric resistance to oxfendazole by nematodes in cattle. Vet Rec 1996;138:67–8.
[70] Stafford K, Coles GC. Nematode control practices and anthelmintic resistance in dairy calves in the southwest of England. Vet Rec 1999;144:659–61.
[71] Anziani OS, Suarez V, Guglielmone AA, et al. Resistance to benzimidazoles and macrocyclic lactone anthelmintics in cattle nematodes in Argentina. Vet Parasitol 2004;122:303–6.
[72] Michel JF, Lancaster MB, Hong C. *Ostertagia ostertagi* protective immunity in calves. The development in calves of a protective immunity to infection with *Ostertagia ostertagi*. Exp Parasitol 1973;33:179–86.
[73] Almeria S, Canals A, Gomez MT, et al. Characterization of protective immune responses in local lymphoid tissues after drug attenuated infections with *Ostertagia ostertagi*. Vet Parasitol 1998;80:53–64.

[74] Gasbarre LC. *Ostertagia ostertagi:* changes in lymphoid populations in the local lymphoid tissues after primary or secondary infection. Vet Parasitol 1994;55:105–14.
[75] Canals A, Zarlenga DS, Almeria S, et al. Cytokine profile induced by a primary infection with *Ostertagia ostertagi* in cattle. Vet Immunol Immunopathol 1997;58:63–75.
[76] Almeria S, Canals A, Zarlenga DS, et al. Isolation and phenotypic characterization of abomasal mucosal lymphocytes in the course of a primary *Ostertagia ostertagi* infection. Vet Immunol Immunopathol 1997;57:87–98.
[77] Claerebout E, Vercauteren I, Geldhof P, et al. Cytokine responses in immunized and non-immunized calves after *Ostertagia* ostertagi infection. Parasite Immunol 2005;27(9):325–31.
[78] Gasbarre LC. Effects of gastrointestinal nematode infection on the ruminant immune system. Vet Parasitol 1997;72:327–43.
[79] Yang C, Gibbs HC, Xiao L. Immunologic changes in *Ostertagia ostertagi*-infected calves treated strategically with an anthelmintic. Am J Vet Res 1993;54:1074–83.
[80] Baker DG, Stott JL, Gershwin LJ. Abomasal lymphatic lymphocyte subpopulations in cattle infected with *Ostertagia* ostertagi and *Cooperia* sp. Vet Immunol Immunopathol 1993; 39:467–73.
[81] Gasbarre LC, Canals A. Induction of protective immunity in calves immunized with adult Oesophagostomum radiatum somatic antigens. Vet Parasitol 1989;34:223–38.
[82] Gasbarre LC, Leighton EA, Davies CJ. Genetic control of immunity to gastrointestinal nematodes of cattle. Vet Parasitol 1990;37:257–72.
[83] Stear MJ, Hetzel DJS, Brown SC, et al. The relationships among ecto- and endoparasite levels, class I antigens of the bovine major histocompatibility system, immunoglobulin E levels and weight gain. Vet Parasitol 1990;34:303–21.
[84] Crofton HD. A quantitative approach to parasitism. Parasitol 1971a;62:179–93.
[85] Crofton HD. A model of host-parasite relationships. Parasitol 1971b;63:343–64.
[86] Genchi C, Madonna M, Traldi G. Epidemiology of *Ostertagia ostertagi* in dairy cow from different breeding systems. Parasitologia 1989;31:123–32.
[87] Gasbarre LC, Leighton EA, Davies CJ. Influence of host genetics upon antibody responses against gastrointestinal nematode infections in cattle. Vet Parasitol 1993;46:81–91.
[88] Anderson RM, May RM. Herd immunity to helminth infection and implications for parasite control. Nature 1985;315:493–6.
[89] Gasbarre LC, Leighton EA, Bryant D. Reliability of a single fecal egg per gram determination as a measure of individual and herd values for trichostrongyle nematodes of cattle. Am J Vet Res 1996;57:168–71.
[90] Leighton EA, Murrell KD, Gasbarre LC. Evidence for genetic control of nematode egg-shedding rates in calves. J Parasitol 1989;75:498–504.
[91] Gasbarre LC, Leighton EA, Bryant D. Genetically controlled resistance to gastrointestinal nematode infections of cattle. Proc Beef Improv Fed 1995;212–7.
[92] Gasbarre LC. Do fecal egg counts accurately reflect worm numbers in cattle? Practical Animal Health, Pfizer Animal Health; 1997. p. 22–7.
[93] Eysker M, Ploeger HW. Value of present diagnostic methods for gastrointestinal nematode infections in cattle. Parasitol 2000;120:109–19.
[94] Claerebout E, Vercruysse J. The immune response and the evaluation of acquired immunity against gastrointestinal nematodes in cattle: a review. Parasitol 2000;120:25–42.
[95] Bryan RP, Kerr JD. The relation between the natural worm burden of steers and the faecal egg count differentiation to species. Vet Parasitol 1989;30:327–34.
[96] Ketzis JK, Vercruysse J, Stromberg BE, et al. Establishing performance requirements for novel methods of controlling helminth infections in ruminants. Vet Parasitol 2006;139: 321–35.
[97] Waller PJ, Thamsborg SM. Nematode control in 'green' ruminant production systems. Trends Parasitol 2004;20:493–7.
[98] Larsen M. Prospect for controlling animal parasitic nematodes by predacious micro fungi. Parasitol 2000;120:S121–31.

[99] Fernández AS, Larsen M, Henningsen E, et al. Effect of *Duddingtonia flagrans* against *Ostertagia ostertagi* in cattle grazing under different stocking rates. Parasitol 1999;119:105–11.

[100] Waller PJ, Schwan O, Ljungstrom BL, et al. Evaluation of biological control of sheep parasites using *Duddingtonia flagrans* under commercial farming conditions on the island of Gotland, Sweden. Vet Parasitol 2004;126:299–315.

[101] Fontenot ME, Miller JE, Pena MT, et al. Efficiency of feeding *Duddingtonia flagrans* chlamydospores to grazing ewes on reducing availability of parasitic nematode larvae on pasture. Vet Parasitol 2003;118:203–13.

[102] Athanasiadou S, Kyriazakis I, Jackson F, et al. Direct anthelmintic effects of condensed tannis towards different gastrointestinal nematodes of sheep: *in vitro* and *in vivo* studies. Vet Parasitol 2001;99:205–19.

[103] Marley CL, Cook R, Keatinge R, et al. The effect of birdsfoot trefoil (*Lotus corniculatus*) and chicory (*Chichorium intybus*) on parasite intensities and performance of lambs naturally infected with helminth parasites. Vet Parasitol 2003;112:147–55.

[104] Stepek G, Behnke JM, Buttle DJ, et al. Natural plant cysteine proteinases as anthelmintics? Trends Parasitol 2004;20:322–7.

[105] Tagboto S, Townson S. Antiparasitic properties of medicinal plants and other naturally occurring products. Adv Parasitol 2001;50:199–295.

[106] Bang KS, Familton AS, Sykes AR. Effect of copper oxide wire particle treatment on establishment of major gastrointestinal nematodes in lambs. Res Vet Sci 1990;49:132–7.

[107] Knox MR. Effectiveness of copper oxide wire particles for *Haemonchus contortus* in sheep. Aust Vet J 2002;80:224–7.

[108] Waller PJ, Bernes G, Rudby-Martin L, et al. Evaluation of copper supplementation to control parasite infections of sheep in Sweden. Svensk Veterinartidning 2004;56:11–6.

[109] Dimander S-O, Höglund J, Waller PJ. Seasonal translation of infective larvae of gastrointestinal nematodes of cattle and the effect of *Duddingtonia flagrans*: a 3-year plot study. Vet Parasitol 2003;117:99–116.

[110] Fernandez MI, Woodward BW, Stromberg BE. Effect of organic and conventional anthelmintics on internal parasites and feedlot performance of beef steers. An Sci 1998;66:635–41.

[111] Bowen FL. Nematode parasite control in weaner cattle on the Northern Tablelands of New South Wales. Aust J Exp Agric Anim Husb 1979;19:269–75.

ELSEVIER
SAUNDERS

Vet Clin Food Anim
22 (2006) 567–581

VETERINARY
CLINICS
Food Animal Practice

Anthelmintic Resistance and Alternative Control Methods

Thomas M. Craig, DVM, PhD

Department of Veterinary Pathobiology, Texas A&M University, College Station, TX 77843-4467, USA

Nematode parasites are economically important in intensive grazing systems. Therefore, livestock producers and veterinarians rely heavily on anthelmintics to eliminate infections and disease, while often ignoring such essential management practices as sanitation and nutrition. Most anthelmintics are safe, efficacious, and broad spectrum in activity; however, the specific nematode, stage of development, and residual activity for which the drug is effective are variable. In general, parasite infections are reduced or eliminated in a flock or herd by anthelmintics. However, even if all parasites were amenable to treatment, and there were sufficient personnel and money available to treat all parasitized animals, this approach would not necessarily eradicate parasites. Anthelmintics can and do save lives and increase profitability. They may also interfere with the ability of the host to mount an effective immunologic response to the very parasites they are used to control. Selection for resistance will inevitably occur when drugs used in attempts to lower parasite levels are not 100% effective, because the survivors have some characteristic that enables them to survive when others die. Clinically relevant resistance is established in a herd, at least in part, by the frequency of treatment. A direct correlation appears to exist between the frequency of anthelmintic administration and the onset of clinical resistance. Anthelmintic resistance has become a major problem in small ruminants in the southern United States.

Anthelmintic treatment to lower levels of infection and increase productivity began with the introduction of thiabendazole in 1961, which was a safe and effective drug. However, resistance by *Haemonchus contortus* was reported in North America by 1964 [1,2] and rapidly spread [3–6]. Despite the lack of exposure to benzimidizole compounds under pasture conditions, populations of thiabendazole-resistant *Haemonchus* were still resistant to

E-mail address: tcraig@cvm.tamu.edu

doi:10.1016/j.cvfa.2006.07.003 **vetfood.theclinics.com**

this class of anthelmintics 15 years later, indicating that there was no reversion to susceptibility under field conditions [7]. Levamisole/morantel resistance [8–10] was reported in the 1980s, followed by resistance to ivermectin [11,12]. Since that time, resistance has increased to the point where no populations of *H contortus* extant in the southern United States are likely to be susceptible to all families of anthelmintics [13–15]. Attempts to evade the problem have involved the use of new drugs effective against resistant parasite populations, such as moxidectin [16,17], or of combinations of drugs [18–20]. However, resistance to all classes of anthelmintics is widespread, as seen in field observations and laboratory studies. Resistance by *Teladorsagia* (*Ostertagia*) and *Trichostrongylus* is documented in small ruminants in Australia, New Zealand, Europe, southern South America, South Africa, and possibly the northern United States.

Numerous studies have compared anthelmintic-resistant and susceptible populations of *Haemonchus*. Various mechanisms are associated with resistance, such as beta-tubulin in benzimidazoles [21], propionyl esterase [22], and P-glycoprotein gene differences in ivermectin resistance [23–26]. In studies with the free-living nematode *Caenorhabditis elegans*, mutation of three genes associated with a glutamate-gated chloride channel was necessary to produce resistance to ivermectin [27]. It is not known whether this is the case with strains of *Haemonchus*, because there appear to be differences among the mechanisms of resistance exhibited by different populations of worms [28–30]. At least some of the resistance seen when multifamily anthelmintic resistance has been identified is associated with P-glycoprotein efflux of the drugs across cell membranes [31]. Biochemical analysis of the expression of susceptible and resistant strains has led to confusion when it comes to consistent identification of resistant populations. However, laboratory models (eg, egg hatch, larval development) are useful in detecting resistance to anthelmintics in populations before clinical disease occurs [32].

The confusion in genetic studies is most likely due to the tremendous diversity seen in *Haemonchus* populations. *H contortus* has such a rich genome that some individuals in a population may have genes to resist the effects of anthelmintics [33,34]. Tolerant or resistant worms accompany livestock introduced to a new farm. The worms accompanying their hosts are likely already to be resistant, so clinical disease develops more rapidly than it would where there are still susceptible worms. Other factors besides the *Haemonchus* genome contribute to the rapid onset of resistance in small ruminants. When underdosing exposes worms to a less than lethal level of anthelmintic, the result is a larger population of survivor worms with a level of resistance. The rapid onset and widespread occurrence of resistance support the contention that selection by treatment and not mutation is the driving force in the establishment of resistance [35]. Given the extreme fecundity of *Haemonchus* and the uneven distribution of larvae in pastures, an individual animal can serve as the nidus for the establishment of resistance on a farm [36], and resistant worms can rapidly become the dominant population.

Resistance to most anthelmintics does not appear to be controlled by a single gene [33]. Underdosing is a powerful selection mechanism for resistance. If the average weight is used to determine the dose for all the animals in the flock or herd, then an underdose is administered to the larger animals. These larger animals may have no signs of disease, but the worms produced in them may have been selected toward resistance. Another way of underdosing is using the same dose in different host species. Goats are able to metabolize anthelmintics more efficiently than cattle [37], and the exposure of worms to ivermectin is four to five times lower in goats than in cattle given the same dose [38]. Another practice that results in underdosing is the subcutaneous use of cattle dewormers in small ruminants [11]. In this case the blood levels are initially high, then drop off. This pattern yields long residual levels, which kill incoming worms for a week to a month or more following the drug's use. In small ruminants, and to a lesser extent in cattle, as the levels drop a few days to a week after treatment, the drug removes only those worms without alleles for resistance [39]. It is a cutting gate, turning back the susceptible and allowing the super worms to establish. The sheep and goat industry did an excellent job of selecting for ivermectin resistance with this practice.

Anthelmintic resistance has been reported in cattle in the United Kingdom [40], New Zealand [41], and Argentina [42], associated with intensively grazed pastures. The reports of anthelmintic resistance in North America are associated with calves grazed similarly. Stocker calves grazed on permanent pastures during the rapid-growth phase of their lives were heavily parasitized, despite prophylactic treatment.

The situation in the United States is most likely due to the normal flow of calves from weaning to the feedlot. The number of calves from a single source is not sufficient to harvest the forage from large pastures, so background operations fulfill this task, collecting calves from many sources. The background operations obtain calves from sale barns in lots ranging from 1 to 100 or more. The calves are then selected by weight, phenotype, age, and sex and placed in groups with their cohorts. They are weaned, vaccinated, given an anthelmintic, introduced to a feed trough, and possibly treated for disease. These calves are under tremendous stress and are exposed to a variety of infectious agents. Often the background calves are maintained on small pastures, which help lessen exposure to respiratory disease but do not provide sufficient forage for their dietary needs. The pastures are seeded with eggs from calves whose parasites were not completely removed on arrival. The larvae from these eggs contaminate the overgrazed pastures and are ingested by susceptible calves. The calves only remain at the backgrounder's for a few weeks or months and seldom show any sign of clinical disease. They then go to the stocker operation, where they are again given an anthelmintic (often the same one as when they arrived at the backgrounder's). A few months into the grazing period, they may show signs of disease caused by the progeny of the resistant worm population obtained from the backgrounder's pasture [43].

Most recent reports of suspected resistance have involved resistance of *Cooperia* and *Nematodirus* to macrocyclic lactones. Ever since this class of drugs was introduced, these parasites have been tolerant of macrolides, so resistance is expected. But both worm genera also stimulate an early protective immune response, and, unless numbers are tremendously high, they are of limited economic importance. The real concern in cattle is reported resistance of *Haemonchus* to macrocyclic lactones and benzimidazoles [43,44]. The history fits the management outlined earlier, and other similar situations have been reported, though without sufficient documentation.

Determination of anthelmintic resistance is often made after a drug fails and animals die or develop severe clinical signs. Clinical response to an anthelmintic occurs with only 40% to 50% efficacy, but this leads to massive pasture build-up of resistant worms, and numbers win. The fecal egg count reduction test (FECRT) is the most common method of evaluating anthelmintic effectiveness in a herd or flock [45]. The evaluation is directed toward strongylate eggs that are similar enough that they cannot reliably be differentiated. The host population and time of year may be useful in determining which eggs will be seen in a given geographic location, but that prediction is not a certainty.

Egg hatch or larval development assays, in which nematode eggs are placed in a solution containing various concentrations of anthelmintics, evaluate the ability of the worms to develop to the infective stage. Some drugs inhibit the ability of the eggs to hatch, others the ability of larvae to feed and molt. The percentages of eggs that are able to develop to infective third-stage larvae are compared with those of eggs not exposed to anthelmintics under identical conditions. Small populations of resistant worms can be detected by this system. Molecular diagnosis using polymerase chain reaction tests has been developed for benzimidazole resistance. The resistance alleles for different species of worm vary, so tests for resistance are not universal, but the approach is promising [46]. Whenever in vitro tests are used, the host species must be considered, because of the variability in pharmacodynamics. In vitro tests should be compared with the FECRT to determine that a sufficient dose was administered appropriately to that population of animals.

When resistance is diagnosed, the worms remain resistant. Benzimidazole-resistant *H contortus* is truly a super worm. It drinks more blood, lays more eggs, and appears to survive longer in the environment [47]. However, not all populations appear to have this inherent advantage over susceptible worms [48]. Levamisole resistance to *Trichostrongylus colubriformis* is a sex-linked recessive resistance factor [49]. Therefore, when levamisole resistance is detected, avoidance of the product for 3 to 6 years may yield a clinically susceptible worm population. Ivermectin-resistant strains of *Haemonchus* appear not to survive as well as susceptible worms during the free-living stages [50]. Ivermectin-resistant larvae do not survive as long at refrigerator temperatures as other populations, which may be a reason why ivermectin resistance is not seen as frequently in the northern United States. This finding may be another reason to treat small ruminants for *Haemonchus* during the winter hypobiotic period.

Management to increase the efficacy of anthelmintics

Benzimidazoles delivered over several days have enhanced efficacy [50–52]. That is, the dose divided and delivered over 3 to 5 days is much more effective against worm populations. A good strategy for deworming livestock involves incorporating the drug in palatable feed and making sure that animals in the herd that require treatment have access to it. The use of blocks or minerals to administer drugs has been disappointing, because the consumption is too variable to ensure that all hosts have adequate daily intake. This hit-or-miss process is likely to lead to low-dose selection for resistance. Overnight fasting before the administration of oral anthelmintics increases the effectiveness of some anthelmintics [53–55]. Fenbendazole, which has low solubility, has increased efficacy when it is administered into the rumen. Rumen fluid increases the amount of active metabolite absorbed and consequently available to worms. However, albendazole, a more soluble compound, has greater efficacy when delivered to the abomasum [56]. With a related compound, oxfendazole, it appears to make no difference whether it is delivered to the rumen or abomasum [57].

When a place where multiple anthelmintic resistance occurs has been identified, combinations of anthelmintics from different families may be the only choice. Even when individual anthelmintics are ineffective, combining drugs may be clinically effective [18–20,58,59]. Various combinations of drugs have been investigated, but it is essential that full therapeutic dosages of each anthelmintic are used and that they are used concurrently. This approach is employed commercially in Australia in the summer rainfall areas; the product currently used is a combination of albendazole, ivermectin, and levamisole. Of course, this approach may have a limited life-span of efficacy, because worms with resistance to each compound are present and will mate to produce multiresistant worms.

The "obvious" way to prevent selection for resistance is to switch the families of anthelmintics used, rotating drugs. Unfortunately, the obvious is wrong: rotation of drugs within a grazing season selects for resistance to all the drugs in the rotation. This process occurs with different drugs at different time intervals but ensures that multiple resistances will develop more rapidly than they would if the drug were used until no longer effective and then switched [19,60]. Yearly rotation may work, because the worms at the beginning of the year are the survivors of last year's treatment regimen and may be susceptible to next year's, and this process does not preselect for resistance to another product. However, the practice of using a product until it fails, then using one from a different family appears to be the best approach [19].

Management to preserve the efficacy of anthelmintics

Targeted deworming, that is treating only the animals at risk [61,62] or individuals with signs of disease (pale mucous membranes, high egg counts, hypoproteinemia), lessens the chances of selecting resistant parasites, because the worms in the untreated animals will survive whether they possess resistant genes or not. The selection of heavily parasitized individuals is labor intensive and requires frequent observation. The FAMACHA approach, named with an acronym for the originator, involves evaluating ocular mucous membrane color with a color chart to determine which individual animals are anemic [63,64]. This methodology is effective where *Haemonchus* is the predominant helminth. The idea is to

- Determine the individual animals that have the largest numbers of worms and selectively treat them, because 20% to 30% of the flock contains 80% of the worms [65]. This method removes most of the sources of pasture contamination but puts no selective pressure on the worms in the remainder of the flock, the refugia worms.
- Evaluate the flock to see how things are going before clinical signs are seen. Animals with various levels of anemia will be identified and a flock score may be kept to observe how the flock in general is doing. Even if the producer decides to treat the entire flock, the treatment will only be administered when needed (a form of tactical treatment), so that less anthelmintic is used and lower pressure is placed on the worm population.
- Improve the genetic resistance of the flock [65]. Resistance to infection with *H contortus* measured by fecal egg count (FEC) and packed cell volume (PCV) is heritable. The same animals tend to exhibit the highest FEC and lowest PCV each time they are measured [66,67]. Removing the most susceptible animals each year will have the long-term effect of improving the overall genetic resistance or resilience of the flock to *H contortus*.

The greatest problem with the FAMACHA approach in the southern United States is the lack of susceptible worms on many pastures.

Nematode parasites of sheep and goats are largely shared. However, the disease exhibited and the management of the infection differ sufficiently that simply substituting "goat" for "sheep" will not tell the entire story. Goats are more selective in their daily foraging and prefer browse to forbs or grass when they have the opportunity. Where sheep and goats cohabit arid rangelands, *Haemonchus* is most often a problem in sheep where the goats have available browse. In other areas, where goats are forced to graze, they are more susceptible to worms and often suffer from disease. Goats metabolize anthelmintics differently from sheep [68,69], and resistance is seen in goats before it is in sheep. Therefore, a 1.5 to 4 times larger dose is necessary to achieve the bioequivalent in the control of parasites [38]. Anthelmintic resistance often begins in goats, then follows in sheep. A likely explanation is that goats metabolize the drugs so rapidly that the worm is exposed to a less than lethal dose, resulting in a higher chance of somewhat resistant worms' mating and being selected further. In the southern United States, *Haemonchus* populations resistant to anthelmintics in goats are the rule.

Resistant worms are purchased in a host that has been treated with an anthelmintic that removed the competition. Maintaining newly purchased animals in a barn or dry lot until they have been evaluated 2 weeks after treatment with an effective combination of anthelmintics is an essential part of a herd's health management [70]. Perhaps the most valuable contribution veterinarians can make to their clients is urging them to remove resistant worms before the pastures become heavily laden.

Management practices to lessen parasite exposure

Lessening exposure of susceptible hosts is paramount in control programs, but one approach will not serve all situations. Each worm species has limitations on its development and survival in the pasture. Warm season parasites, such as *Haemonchus*, are readily transmitted during the summer but become quiescent on pasture during the cool season and are unlikely to ascend the vegetation and be acquired during grazing. Cool season parasites may be transmitted all winter in the south but die quickly in summer pastures. When worms enter the host, they molt and become adult worms that begin producing eggs approximately 3 weeks after acquisition from the pasture. When larvae acquired during transitional seasons became adults, their offspring are subject to an unfavorable environment, so incoming larvae undergo arrested development (hypobiosis) within the host. During hypobiosis, worms suspend their development and remain immature in the host's digestive tract [71]. During this period of hypobiosis, they do not feed, lay eggs, or in any way cause damage to the host. Because they are inactive, the host is unable to recognize their presence, and even if the host has the capacity to protect itself from worms it is unable to do so. When environmental conditions change and or the host's immunity wanes, larvae resume development en masse. This development may cause clinical disease when the numbers are sufficient. Parasite numbers are important, but the number that is clinically significant varies greatly with the host and parasite species.

The most important parasite of small ruminants in the southern United States is *H contortus,* which undergoes winter arrest. Larvae acquired in pasture in many areas during September and October arrest until the ewe or doe gives birth or spring arrives. When the larvae become active, they rapidly mature and begin egg production. The eggs produced from formerly arrested, now active worms and the larvae that survived in the pasture overwinter are now available for transmission to the adult animals and their offspring [9]. Transmission begins with the sustained growth of warm season forage. Larvae on the pasture during the winter are inactive, and many perish during a dry winter by desiccation. In humid areas, they become active when the weather begins to warm up, but they only survive for a short time before their stored energy is depleted. In a similar manner, the most important cattle parasite, *Ostertagia ostertag*, undergoes summer arrest in the southern United States. *Ostertagia* larvae rapidly perish in summer pastures, especially when there are rains to break up the fecal pats. Arrested *Ostertagia* larvae become active during the autumn and provide eggs for the winter and spring pastures.

Evading larvae in pastures by removing livestock to render a pasture parasite-safe may be accomplished in 1 month in a warm, wet summer but may take as long as 8 months in a cool, humid climate. Management systems that lower the exposure of hosts to parasites by long-term vacating of pastures may be counterproductive, because the forage from the vacated pasture is overly mature, with low palatability and protein content. By contrast, high-density, short-duration rotation systems may increase the level of parasite exposure but optimize the value of forages, resulting in healthier livestock because of a better nutritional plane. In humid, tropical climates, rapid rotation, in which pastures are vacated for as few as 30 days, lowers larval numbers significantly [72]. Using pastures that have been used for cropping, especially in the last half of the grazing season, is an effective measure for reducing challenge. Alternate or cograzing by hosts of a different class or species may lower exposure when the target animals return to the pasture. In general, *Haemonchus* of sheep and goats do not do well in cattle, and vice versa. However, some populations of *H contortus* may thrive in calves [73].

Although anthelmintics are important in eliminating helminths from the host, good-quality nutritious feed is equally important to the health and well-being of parasitized animals. Most clinical helminthiasis occurs in hosts that exist on marginal rations. None of the anthelmintics will increase the weight gain of an animal unless adequate rations are available. Providing sufficient dietary protein is vital during the periparturient period and during rapid growth, so that animals will be better able to tolerate the worm burden and will have increased resistance to infection [74]. However, the increased protein found in legumes may or may not affect the establishment of gastrointestinal nematodes [75]. When plants high in condensed tannins are grazed, such as *Sericea lespedeza,* evidence suggests that the incoming larvae are adversely affected, and bypass protein is provided for the host and enhanced immune response [76]. The physical structure of some plants may make it challenging for larvae to ascend vegetation or may provide protection from adverse pasture conditions [77]. When animals are allowed to browse, their chances of acquiring larvae diminish, because the distance from the ground increases, and most infective larvae are found within 50 mm of the soil surface.

A number of influences in a pasture affect the ability of parasitic eggs to hatch and larvae to develop to the infective stage. Earthworms and dung beetles, which may either bury eggs or larvae or affect the dung pat, increasing desiccation, have an effect on survival of parasitic nematodes [78]. Bacterial toxins, such as those produced by *Bacillus thuringiensis,* have a deleterious effect on the development of nematodes in the pasture [79]. Some fungi kill larval nematodes. One species, *Duddingtonia flagrans,* is able to traverse the digestive tract and is present in the fecal pat when larvae hatch. Feeding or incorporating *D flagrans* spores in ruminal boluses suppresses pasture contamination by nematode larvae [80,81].

Nonorganic chemicals used to control parasites, such as copper oxide wire particles, have been shown to protect ewes from *Haemonchus* infections [82]. These may only be used with care in sheep, however, because they are susceptible to chronic copper poisoning. The concurrent use of copper oxide wire and *D flagrans*, when administered early in the grazing season, may have a prolonged effect in terms of lowering pasture contamination as well as increasing the safety margin [83]. For years, livestock owners in various parts of the world have used various botanical products, but few of these have been subjected to scientific scrutiny. Certainly, products containing nicotine, extract of male fern, arecoline, and *Artemisia* spp have all been used with variable success in the control of helminths [84,85]. Problems associated with botanicals include the variability of the active principals at various times in the growth cycle, the influence of differences in climate and soils, and the expectations of the livestock owner. Some of these products may be an alternative to modern anthelmintics, but more research remains to be done before their use becomes widespread.

One apparently logical approach is selection of individual animals with resistance to the parasite or those that have the capacity to rebound from the effects of parasitism. The offspring of resistant hosts are likely to be resistant. Therefore, resistance to *Haemonchus* or other locally important parasites should be a selection criterion used in flocks [86–92]. Features such as the effect of CD4+ T cells on the expression of resistance indicate its importance in the mediation of resistance [93]. An increase in serum IgG1 and IgA levels is associated with genetically resistant sheep [94]. Likewise, the number of IgE-bearing cells may be associated with the capability of the host to respond to helminth infection [95].

The genetic aspect of resistance to gastrointestinal parasites is not well understood. It appears that multiple genes are involved in the protective response and that different genes may be more important at various times in the course of infection and to infection by different species of worms [96]. To some extent, in all breeds, some individual animals possess resistance factors that make them more likely to survive exposure levels that would severely affect other animals. Even in resistant breeds all animals are not equal, and factors such as lactation, age, and nutritional status may influence the course of disease. When animals are producing at their genetic maximum, they are at greatest risk for parasitic disease because they are immunologically or nutritionally challenged or both [97]. Other phenotypic characteristics, such as production of milk, fiber, multiple births, and resistance to other agents, may be at odds with resistance to helminths. Research does not indicate that the traits that lead to increased production are linked to those of increased susceptibility or resistance.

Acquired resistance to parasitism strongly indicates that vaccines against parasitic nematodes should be an effective approach to control. However, this approach has met with disappointment: the hosts with the genetic potential to resist the parasites were aided, but the susceptible hosts remained at risk. Another approach is the use of cryptic antigens (from parasite intestinal cells that do not contact the host immune-processing cells), which are injected into hosts so that, when the parasite takes a blood meal, the antibody formed acts to destroy the parasite's gut cells [98,99]. This approach may become useful when an inexpensive way of producing sufficient amounts of antigen is developed.

The most important factor in control is knowing whether the anthelmintic that was administered actually worked. Clinical response is not sufficient. Response should be judged by a larval development assay or fecal egg reduction trial at each and every farm that has small ruminants. When anthelmintic resistance is encountered, the failed drug should only be used on that farm against other parasite species as necessary, because the likelihood of the target species' becoming susceptible to the specific drug is low.

In the early spring or at the onset of the rainy season, reduced pasture contamination is most important. Ewes or does in the periparturient relaxation of resistance, even those that have the genetic capacity for resistance, are a source of eggs for the environment. Strategic deworming to remove arrested or recently emerged larvae before they contaminate the pasture has a great impact on subsequent pasture exposure [9,100,101]. Worms survive by sheer numbers, avoiding unfavorable conditions in the environment by undergoing arrested development or surviving in fecal pats; evading host immune response through arrested development or intermittent exposure. They reproduce during the periparturient period in young hosts. Worms also have a broad genetic base so that, when environmental conditions change, there are survivors that can adjust to the new conditions or tolerate anthelmintics to which they have never been exposed. The offspring of tolerant worms become resistant and rapidly predominate as the less fit individuals are removed by anthelmintics.

References

[1] Drudge JH, Szato J, Wyant ZN, et al. Studies on parasite control in sheep: comparison of thiabendazole, rulene, and phenothiazine. Am J Vet Res 1964;25:1513–8.

[2] Conway DP. Variance in the effectiveness of thiabendazole against *Haemonchus contortus* in sheep. Am J Vet Res 1964;25:844–5.
[3] Shelton M. An evaluation of some newer anthelmintics. J Anim Sci 1968;27:1136.
[4] Anderson FL, Christofferson PV. Efficacy of haloxon and thiabendazole against gastrointestinal nematodes in sheep and goats in the Edwards plateau area of Texas. Am J Vet Res 1973;34:1395–8.
[5] Miller JE, Baker NF. Thiabendazole-resistant strains of *Haemonchus* and *Ostertagia* in California lambs. Am J Vet Res 1980;41:1674–6.
[6] Uhlinger C, Fetrow J, Johnstone C. A field evaluation of benzimidazole and nonbenzimidazole drugs in a herd of dairy goats. J Vet Intern Med 1988;2:113–6.
[7] Lyons ET, Drudge JH, Tolliver SC, et al. Controlled tests on activity of contemporary parasiticides on natural infections of helminths in lambs, with emphasis on strains of *Haemonchus contortus* isolated in 1955. Am J Vet Res 1992;53:91–6.
[8] Hembry FG, Miller JE, Sims D, et al. Efficacy of repeated doses of levamisole, morantel, fenbendazole, and ivermectin against gastrointestinal nematodes in ewes. Am J Vet Res 1986;47:1677–9.
[9] Craig TM. Epidemiology and control of gastrointestinal nematodes and cestodes in small ruminants: southern United States. Vet Clin North Am Food Anim Pract 1986;2:367–72.
[10] Miller JE, Hembry FG, Kearney MT, et al. Efficacy of levamisole and netobimin against *Haemonchus contortus* in lambs in Louisiana. Am J Vet Res 1987;48:1403–6.
[11] Craig TM, Miller DK. Resistance by *Haemonchus contortus* to ivermectin in Angora goats. Vet Rec 1990;126:580.
[12] Miller JE, Barras SR. Ivermectin resistant *Haemonchus contortus* in Louisiana lambs. Vet Parasitol 1994;55:343–6.
[13] Zajac AM, Gipson TA. Multiple anthelmintic resistance in a goat herd. Vet Parasitol 2000; 87:163–72.
[14] Mortensen LL, Williamson LH, Terrill TT, et al. Evaluation of prevalence and clinical implications of anthelmintic resistance in gastrointestinal nematodes in goats. J Am Vet Med Assoc 2003;223:495–500.
[15] Kaplan RM. Drug resistance in nematodes of veterinary importance: a status report. Trends Parasitol 2004;20:477–81.
[16] Craig TM, Hatfield TA, Pankavich JA, et al. Efficacy of moxidectin against an ivermectin resistant strain of *Haemonchus contortus* in sheep. Vet Parasitol 1992;41: 329–33.
[17] Pankavitch JA, Berger H, Simkins KL. Efficacy of moxidectin, nemadectin and ivermectin against an ivermectin-resistant strain of *Haemonchus contortus* in sheep. Vet Rec 1992;130: 241–3.
[18] Anderson N, Martin PJ, Jarrett RG. The efficacy of mixtures of albendazole sulphoxides and levamisole against sheep nematodes resistant to benzimidazole and levamisole. Aust Vet J 1991;68:127–32.
[19] Barnes EH, Dobson RJ, Barger IA. Worm control and anthelmintic resistance: adventures with a model. Parasitol Today 1995;11:56–63.
[20] Miller DK, Craig TM. Use of anthelmintic combinations against multiple resistant *Haemonchus contortus* in Angora goats. Small Rumin Res 1996;19:281–3.
[21] Lubega GW, Prichard RK. Beta-tubulin and benzimidazole resistance in the sheep nematode *Haemonchus contortus*. Mol Biochem Parasitol 1991;47:129–38.
[22] Echevarria FAM, Gennari SM, Tait A. Isoenzyme analysis of *Haemonchus contortus* resistant or susceptible to ivermectin. Vet Parasitol 1992;44:87–95.
[23] Xu M, Molento M, Blackhall W, et al. Ivermectin resistance in nematodes may be caused by alteration of P-glycoprotein homolog. Mol Biochem Parasitol 1998;91:327–35.
[24] Blackhall WJ, Liu HY, Xu M, et al. Selection at a P-glycoprotein gene in ivermectin- and moxidectin-selected strains of *Haemonchus contortus*. Mol Biochem Parasitol 1998;95: 193–201.

[25] Blackhall WJ, Pouliot J-F, Prichard RK, et al. *Haemonchus contortus*: selection at a glutamate-gated chloride channel gene in ivermectin- and moxidectin-selected strains. Exp Parasitol 1998;90:42–8.
[26] von Samson-Himmelstjerna G, Blackhall W. Will technology provide solutions for drug resistance in veterinary helminths? Vet Parasitol 2005;132:223–39.
[27] Dent JA, Smith MM, Vassilatis DK, et al. The genetics of ivermectin resistance in *Caenorhabditis elegans*. Proc Natl Acad Sci U S A 2000;97:2674–9.
[28] Gill JH, Lacey E. Avermectin/milbemycin resistant trichostrongyloid nematodes. Int J Parasitol 1998;28:863–77.
[29] Gill JH, Kerr CA, Shoop WL, et al. Evidence of multiple mechanisms of avermectin resistance in *Haemonchus contortus*—comparison of selection protocols. Int J Parasitol 1998;28: 783–9.
[30] Wolstenholme AJ, Fairweather I, Prichard R, et al. Drug resistance in veterinary helminths. Trends Parasitol 2004;20:469–76.
[31] Kerboeuf D, Guegnard F, Le Vern Y. Analysis and partial reversal of multidrug resistance to anthelmintics due to P-glycoprotein in *Haemonchus contortus* eggs using *Lens culinaris* lectin. Parasitol Res 2002;88:816–21.
[32] Maingi N, Bjorn H, Dangolla A. The relationship between fecal egg count reduction and the lethal dose 50% in the egg hatch assay and larval development assay. Vet Parasitol 1998;77:133–45.
[33] Otsen M, Hoekstra R, Plas ME, et al. Amplified fragment length polymorphism analysis of genetic diversity of *Haemonchus contortus* during selection for drug resistance. Int J Parasitol 2001;31:1138–43.
[34] Prichard R. Genetic variability following selection of *Haemonchus contortus* with anthelmintics. Trends Parasitol 2001;17:445–53.
[35] Smith G, Grenfell BT, Isham V, et al. Anthelmintic resistance revisited: under-dosing, chemoprophylactic strategies, and mating probabilities. Int J Parasitol 1999;29: 77–91.
[36] Cornell SJ, Isham VS, Smith G, et al. Spatial parasite transmission, drug resistance, and the spread of rare genes. Proc Natl Acad Sci U S A 2003;100:7401–5.
[37] Scott EW, Kinabo LD, Mckeller QA. Pharmacokinetics of ivermectin after oral administration to adult milking goats. J Vet Pharmacol Ther 1990;13:432–5.
[38] Gonzalez A, Sahagun AM, Diez MJ, et al. Pharmacokinetics of a novel formulation of ivermectin after administration to goats. Am J Vet Res 2006;67:323–8.
[39] Lespine A, Alvinerie M, Sutra J-F, et al. Influence of the route of administration on efficacy and tissue distribution of ivermectin in goats. Vet Parasitol 2005;128:251–60.
[40] Coles GC, Watson CL, Anziani OS. Ivermectin-resistant *Cooperia* in cattle. Vet Rec 2001; 148:283–4.
[41] Familton AS, Mason P, Coles GC. Anthelmintic resistant *Cooperia* in New Zealand cattle. Vet Rec 2001;149:719–20.
[42] Anziani OS, Suarez V, Guglielmone AA, et al. Resistance to benzimidazole and macrocyclic lactone anthelmintics in cattle nematodes in Argentina. Vet Parasitol 2004;122: 303–6.
[43] Gasbarre LC, Smith LL, Lichtenfels JR, et al. The identification of cattle nematode parasites resistant to multiple classes of anthelmintics in a commercial cattle population in the US. Proc Am Assoc Vet Parasitol 2004;49:44.
[44] Gasbarre LC, Smith LL, Pilitt PA. Identification of cattle nematodes resistant to multiple classes of anthelmintics in a commercial cattle population in the US. Proc Am Assoc Vet Parasitol 2005;50:46.
[45] Coles GC, Jackson F, Pomroy WE, et al. The detection of anthelmintic resistance in nematodes of veterinary importance. Vet Parasitol 2006;136:167–85.
[46] von Samson-Himmelstjerna G. Molecular diagnosis of anthelmintic resistance. Vet Parasitol 2006;136:99–107.

[47] Kelly JD, Whitlock HV, Thompson HG, et al. Physiological characteristics of the free living and parasitic stages of strains of *Haemonchus contortus*, susceptible or resistant to benzimidazole anthelmintics. Res Vet Sci 1978;25:376–85.
[48] Scott EW, Armour J. Effect of development of resistance to benzimidazoles, salicylanilides and ivermectin on the pathogenicity and survival of *Haemonchus contortus*. Vet Rec 1991; 128:346–9.
[49] Martin PJ, McKenzie JA. Levamisole resistance in *Trichostrongylus colubriformis*: a sex-linked recessive character. Int J Parasitol 1990;20:867–72.
[50] Prichard RK, Hennessy DR, Steel JW. Prolonged administration; a new concept for increasing the spectrum and effectiveness of anthelmintics. Vet Parasitol 1978;4: 309–15.
[51] Hass DK, Holliway EL, Brown LJ. Comparison of ruminant anthelmintics using multiple dose administration. Am J Vet Res 1982;43:534–7.
[52] Craig TM. The anthelmintic dilemma. Compendium Continuing Education for the Practicing Veterinarian 1999;21(4 Suppl):S125–43.
[53] Taylor SM, Mallon TR, Blanchflower WJ, et al. Effects of diet on plasma concentrations of oral anthelmintics for cattle and sheep. Vet Rec 1992;130:264–8.
[54] Hennessy DR, Ali DN, Sillince J. The effect of a short term reduction in feed on the pharmacokinetics and efficacy of albendazole in sheep. Aust Vet J 1995;72:29–30.
[55] Ali DN, Hennessy DR. The effect of level of feed intake on the pharmacokinetic disposition and efficacy of ivermectin in sheep. J Pharmacol Ther 1996;19:89–94.
[56] Steel JW, Hennessey DR. Influence of rumen bypass on the pharmacokinetics and efficacy of benzimidazole anthelmintics in sheep. Int J Parasitol 1999;29:305–14.
[57] Sargison ND, Stafford KJ, West DM, et al. The effect of ruminoreticulum bypass in yarded lambs on the efficacy of oxfendazole against resistant *Trichostrongylus* spp helminths. Small Rumin Res 2000;35:213–7.
[58] Waller PJ, Dobson RJ, Haughey KG. The effect of combinations of anthelmintics on parasite populations in sheep. Aust Vet J 1990;67:138–40.
[59] Dobson RJ, Besier RB, Barnes EH, et al. Principles for the use of macrocyclic lactones to minimize selection for resistance. Aust Vet J 2001;79:756–61.
[60] Coles GC. Strategies for control of anthelmintic-resistant nematodes in ruminants. J Am Vet Med Assoc 1988;192:330–4.
[61] Hoste H, LeFrileux Y, Pommaret A. Comparison of selective and systematic treatments to control nematode infection of the digestive tract of dairy goats. Vet Parasitol 2002;106: 345–55.
[62] Hoste H, Chartier C, LeFrileux Y, et al. Targeted application of anthelmintics to control trichostrongylosis in dairy goats; result from a 2-year survey in farms. Vet Parasitol 2002;110:101–8.
[63] van Wyk JA, Bath GF. The FAMACHA(c) system for managing haemonchosis in sheep and goats by clinically identifying individual animals for treatment. Vet Res 2002;33: 509–29.
[64] Sreter T, Molnar V, Kassai T. The distribution of nematode egg counts and larval counts in grazing sheep and their implications for parasite control. Int J Parasitol 1994;24:103–8.
[65] Kaplan RM, Burke JM, Terrill TH, et al. Validation of the FAMACHA(c) eye color chart for detecting clinical anemia in sheep and goats on farms in the southern United States. Vet Parasitol 2004;123:105–20.
[66] Barger IA. The statistical distribution of trichostrongylid nematodes in grazing lambs. Int J Parasitol 1985;15:645–9.
[67] Barger IA, Dash KM. Repeatability of ovine fecal egg counts and blood packed cell volumes in *Haemonchus contortus* infections. Int J Parasitol 1987;17:977–80.
[68] Hall CA, Ritchie L, McDonell PA. Investigations for anthelmintic resistance in gastrointestinal nematodes from goats. Res Vet Sci 1981;31:116–9.

[69] Charlier C, Pors I, Galtier P, et al. Efficacy and pharmacokinetics of levamisole hydrochloride in experimental infections with *Haemonchus contortus* and *Trichostrongylus colubriformis* in dairy goats. J Vet Pharmacol Ther 1997;20(Suppl 1):160.
[70] Fleming SA, Craig T, Kaplan RM, et al. Anthelmintic resistance of gastrointestinal parasites in small ruminants. J Vet Intern Med 2006;20:435–44.
[71] Gibbs HC. Mechanisms of survival of nematode parasites with emphasis on hypobiosis. Vet Parasitol 1982;11:25–48.
[72] Barger IA, Siale K, Banks DJD, et al. Rotational grazing for control of gastrointestinal nematodes of goats in a wet tropical environment. Vet Parasitol 1994;53:109–16.
[73] DeVaney JA, Craig TM, Roe LD. Resistance to ivermectin by *Haemonchus contortus* in goats and calves. Int J Parasitol 1992;22:369–76.
[74] Coop R, Kyriazakis I. Influence of host nutrition on the development and consequences of nematode parasitism in ruminants. Trends Parasitol 2001;17:325–30.
[75] Marley CL, Fraser MD, Fychan R, et al. Effect of forage legumes and anthelmintic treatment on the performance, nutritional status and nematode parasites of grazing lambs. Vet Parasitol 2005;131:267–82.
[76] Min BR, Hart SP, Miller D, et al. The effect of grazing forage containing condensed tannins on gastro-intestinal parasite infection and milk composition in Angora does. Vet Parasitol 2005;130:105–13.
[77] Kates KC. Ecological aspects of helminth transmission in domesticated animals. Am Zool 1965;5:95–130.
[78] Gronvold J, Hendriksen SA, Larsen M, et al. Biological control. Aspects of biological control—with special reference to arthropods, protozoans and helminths of domesticated animals. Vet Parasitol 1996;64:47–64.
[79] Ciordia H, Bizzell WE. A preliminary report on the effects of *Bacillus thuringensis* Berliner on the development of free-living stages of some cattle nematodes. J Parasitol 1961;47:41.
[80] Larsen M. Biological control of helminths. Int J Parasitol 1999;29:139–46.
[81] Waller PJ. Global perspectives on nematode parasite control in ruminant livestock: the need to adopt alternatives to chemotherapy, with emphasis on biological control. Anim Health Res Rev 2003;4:35–43.
[82] Burke JM, Miller JE, Brauer DK. The effectiveness of copper oxide wire particles as an anthelmintic in pregnant ewes and safety of offspring. Vet Parasitol 2005;131:291–7.
[83] Burke JM, Miller JE, Larsen M, et al. Interaction between copper oxide wire particles and *Duddingtonia flagrans* in lambs. Vet Parasitol 2005;134:141–6.
[84] Hammond JA, Fielding D, Bishop SC. Prospects for plant anthelmintics in tropical veterinary medicine. Vet Res Comm 1997;21:213–28.
[85] Alawa CBI, Adamu AM, Gefu JO, et al. In vitro screening of two Nigerian medical plants (*Vernoia amygdalina* and *Annona senegalensis*) for anthelmintic activity. Vet Parasitol 2003; 113:73–81.
[86] Adams DB. Infection with *Haemonchus contortus* in sheep and the role of adaptive immunity in selection of the parasite. Int J Parasitol 1984;18:1071–5.
[87] Courtney CH, Parker CF, McClure KE, et al. A comparison of the periparturient rise in fecal egg counts of exotic and domestic ewes. Int J Parasitol 1984;14:377–81.
[88] Gray GD, Barger IA, LeJambre LF, et al. Parasitological and immunological responses of genetically resistant Merino sheep on pastures contaminated with parasitic nematodes. Int J Parasitol 1992;22:417–25.
[89] Miller JE, Bahirathan M, Lemaire SL, et al. Epidemiology of gastrointestinal nematode parasitism in Suffolk and Gulf Coast native sheep with special emphasis on relative susceptibility to *Haemonchus contortus* infection. Vet Parasitol 1998;74:55–74.
[90] Bisset SA, Morris CA, McEwan JC, et al. Breeding sheep in New Zealand that are less reliant on anthelmintics to maintain health and productivity. N Z Vet J 2001;49(6):236–46.

[91] Amarante AFT, Craig TM, Ramsey WS, et al. Comparison of naturally acquired parasite burdens among Florida native, Rambouillet and crossbreed ewes. Vet Parasitol 1999;85: 61–9.

[92] Notter DR, Andrew SA, Zajac AM. Responses of hair and wool sheep to a single fixed dose of infective larvae of *Haemonchus contortus*. Small Rumin Res 2003;47:221–5.

[93] Gill HS, Watson DL, Brandon MR. Monoclonal antibody to CD4+ T cells abrogates genetic resistance to *Haemonchus contortus* in sheep. Immunology 1993;78:43–9.

[94] Gill HS, Gray GD, Watson DL, et al. Isotype-specific antibody responses to *Haemonchus contortus* in genetically resistant sheep. Parasite Immunol 1993;15:61–7.

[95] Pettit JJ, Jackson F, Rocchi M, et al. The relationship between responsiveness against gastrointestinal nematodes in lambs and the numbers of circulating IgE bearing cells. Vet Parasitol 2005;134:131–9.

[96] Stear MJ, Bishop SC, Mallard BA, et al. The sustainability, feasibility and desirability of breeding livestock for disease resistance. Res Vet Sci 2001;71:1–7.

[97] Bricarello PA, Amarante AFT, Rocha RA, et al. Influence of dietary protein supply on resistance to experimental infections with *Haemonchus contortus* in Ile de France and Santa Ines lambs. Vet Parasitol 2005;134:99–109.

[98] Smith WD. Prospects for vaccines of helminth parasites of grazing ruminants. Int J Parasitol 1999;29:17–24.

[99] Knox D, Smith WD. Vaccination against gastrointestinal nematode parasites of ruminants using gut-expressed antigens. Vet Parasitol 2001;100:21–32.

[100] Darvill FM, Arundel JH, Brown PB. The effect of anthelmintic treatment of maiden ewes in the periparturient period on pasture contamination and production of prime lambs. Aust Vet J 1978;54:575–84.

[101] Herd RP, Streitel RH, McClure KE, et al. Control of periparturient rise in worm egg counts of lambing ewes. J Am Vet Med Assoc 1983;182:375–9.

ELSEVIER
SAUNDERS

Vet Clin Food Anim
22 (2006) 583–593

VETERINARY
CLINICS
Food Animal Practice

Lungworms of Ruminants

Carla Panuska, MS, PhD

College of Veterinary Medicine, Mississippi State University, PO Box 6100, Mississippi State, MS 39762, USA

Ruminants are host to several lungworms that are capable of causing respiratory disease. These include *Dictyocaulus viviparus* in cattle and *Dictyocaulus filaria, Muellerius capillaris,* and *Protostrongylus rufescens* in sheep and goats. Respiratory disease due to infection with these parasites occurs less frequently in North America than in other parts of the world but can be locally or regionally important. Parasitic pneumonia resulting from infection with *D viviparus* has been reported in both beef and dairy cattle in the northern and southern United States [1–3]. Of the small ruminant lungworms, *D filaria* is most pathogenic, whereas infections with *M capillaris* are often inapparent. *D filaria*, like *D viviparus*, is more common in moist climates where the free-living infectious stages can survive. In contrast, transmission of *M capillaris* requires a molluscan intermediate host; however, these parasites are common and have been reported in Canada and the northeastern, northwestern, and southeastern United States [4–7]. *P rufescens* is present worldwide but is not often reported in the United States [8] and is not covered in this discussion.

Dictyocaulus viviparus

The life cycle of *D viviparus* is direct. Adults produce embryonated, thin-shelled eggs that measure 82 to 88 μm by 32 to 38 μm [9]. Eggs hatch shortly after oviposition in the airways or, after being coughed up and swallowed, in the large intestine. First-stage larvae are passed in the feces of the host into the environment, where they can develop to second- and third-stage larvae within a week. The ensheathed third-stage larvae are infective to grazing cattle. Once ingested, the third-stage larvae exsheath in the abomasum, penetrate the intestine, and migrate to the mesenteric lymph nodes near the ileum, cecum, and the proximal colon, where they remain for 3 to 8 days.

E-mail address: panuska@cvm.msstate.edu

0749-0720/06/$ - see front matter
doi:10.1016/j.cvfa.2006.06.002 **vetfood.theclinics.com**

Fourth-stage larvae reach the lungs as early as 7 days after infection and are present in large numbers by 13 to 15 days after infection [10]. The prepatent period is 3 to 4 weeks, though the presence of arrested late fourth-stage larvae or young adults (fifth stage) in the lungs can extend this period to as long as 150 days [11].

Cattle lungworms occur throughout North America, but they are most problematic in moist climates, where pasture larvae are protected from desiccation and migration of the larvae from the fecal pat to herbage is facilitated. Larvae are relatively inactive and are easily trapped within the fecal pat. Heavy rains may scatter larvae, or the larvae may accumulate on the sporangium of the fungus *Pilobolus*, which grows in cattle dung; explosion of the sporangium to disperse fungal spores also propels larvae away from the fecal pat [12]. Mechanical disruption of fecal material may also aid dispersal.

Lungworm disease is seasonal and depends on the availability of infective larvae on pasture. Under favorable conditions, third-stage larvae can survive on pasture for approximately 11 months, overwintering in temperate areas [13,14]. These larvae, combined with larvae shed from carrier animals, serve to contaminate pastures in early spring. Consequently, clinical disease occurs in susceptible calves in late summer or early autumn after several months on pasture. In subtropical climates, such as Louisiana, pasture larvae are most numerous and disease outbreaks most prevalent during the mild winters and early springs; pasture larvae are virtually absent in the hot summers, when carrier animals are an important source of infective larvae for autumn infections [3]. In this area, clinical disease was found to relate to both rainfall and low temperature.

Infection with *D viviparus* can result in parasitic pneumonia and bronchitis; however, infection with few worms may be inapparent. Four phases occur in the development of disease: the penetration phase, the prepatent phase, the patent phase, and the postpatent phase [10,15,16]. The penetration phase, in which there are no clinical signs or significant pathologic conditions, occurs from days 1 to 7 after infection, when larvae are ingested and migrate to the lungs. During the prepatent phase, days 7 to 25, larvae enter the lung tissue and bronchioles; significant signs and pathologic conditions occur. Lesions in the lungs occur as early as 7 days after infection. Respiratory bronchioles are blocked with eosinophilic exudate, excessive mucus is produced, and alveoli collapse; tachypnea and coughing occur, and emphysema is possible. The patent phase, from 25 to 55 days after infection, is associated with the presence of egg-laying adults in the bronchi and trachea. The epithelium of the bronchi and trachea is damaged, air passages are blocked by exudate, and consolidation of lobules results from the aspiration of eggs and first-stage larvae into the brochioles and alveoli. Bronchitis, tracheitis, and pneumonia produce significant clinical signs: dyspnea, coughing, pyrexia, loss of condition, harsh respiratory sounds with rhonchi, and emphysematous crackling. First-stage larvae are abundant in fecal material.

Surviving animals recover during the postpatent phase. The number of adult worms in the bronchi decreases, and few to no larvae are present in the feces. Peribronchial fibrosis and epithelialization of a few alveoli may remain, but the respiratory rate decreases, coughing diminishes, and weight gain resumes. Pulmonary edema, interstitial emphysema, alveolar epithelial hyperplasia, and secondary bacterial infections may complicate the pathologic conditions resulting from infection.

The extent of disease depends on the number of larvae ingested, the rate of ingestion, and the number of larvae reaching the lungs. Disease most often occurs in calves, because cattle rapidly develop an acquired immunity to *D viviparus*. Immunity prevents ingested larvae from establishing, stops development, and eliminates larvae in the lung [17]. Without re-exposure to infective larvae, immunity wanes, and disease can occur in adult cattle when they are exposed to reinfection. However, exposure of immune cattle to large numbers of infective larvae may also result in the "reinfection syndrome." Because of the large numbers of larvae ingested, some escape immune elimination and enter the lungs, causing severe respiratory signs 14 to 16 days after exposure. Severe, frequent coughing, increased respiratory rate, and harsh respiratory sounds without rhonchi and crackling result from an immune reaction in the bronchioles where the larvae are killed. Pulmonary lymphoid nodules 3 to 4 mm in diameter occur under the visceral pleura of the lung, and greenish mucus infiltrated with eosinophils is present in the bronchial tree. Interstitial emphysema and pulmonary edema do not occur. Few or no adult parasites are present; therefore, first-stage larvae are not present in feces.

A number of anthelmintics are available for the treatment and control of *D viviparus* in cattle (Table 1). In addition to being effective against both adult and fourth-stage larvae, the avermectins/milbemycins have demonstrated persistent activity. Moxidectin, ivermectin, doramectin, and eprinomectin are labeled for protection against reinfection for 3 to 6 weeks after treatment, depending on the compound and formulation. Several longer-acting formulations of moxidectin are currently under study; a 1% nonaqueous injectable (0.2 mg/kg) and a long-acting injectable (1.0 mg/kg) provided at least 42 days and 120 days of protection from reinfection, respectively [18,19]. The wide use of effective broad-spectrum anthelmintics such as the benzimidazoles, imidazothiazoles, and avermectin/milbemycins has raised the concern that they may interfere with the natural acquisition of immunity to lungworm infection. Although experimental evidence is sometimes contradictory, anthelmintics, including endectocides, do appear to reduce the acquired immune response compared with that of animals allowed to recover naturally from infection. However, immune protection is still induced in animals treated with these compounds [20–24].

Strategic anthelmintic treatment includes both the prophylactic treatment of susceptible animals to prevent disease and the treatment of carrier animals to prevent contamination of pasture. Additionally, management

Table 1
Approved anthelmintics for treatment and control of *Dictyocaulus* spp in cattle and sheep in the United States

Drug	Dosage[a]	Species (stage)	Preslaughter withdrawal
Fenbendazole	5 mg/kg PO	*D viviparus*	8–16 d[b]
Oxfendazole	4.5 mg/kg PO, intraruminally	*D viviparus* (adult/L4)	7 d
Levamisole	8 mg/kg PO	*D viviparus*	48 h
		D filaria	72 h
	6 mg/kg SC (cattle)	*Dictyocaulus* sp	7 d
	Bolus (cattle)	*Dictyocaulus* sp	48 h
	(sheep)	*Dictyocaulus* sp	72 h
Albendazole	10 mg/kg PO	*D viviparus* (adult and L4)	27 d
	7.5 mg/kg PO	*D filaria* (adult and larval)	7 d
Eprinomectin	0.5 mg/kg pour-on	*D viviparus* (adult/L4)	None
Moxidectin	0.5 mg/kg pour-on	*D viviparus* (adult/L4)	None
	0.2 mg/kg SC	*D viviparus* (adult/L4)	21 d
Doramectin	0.2 mg/kg SC, IM	*D viviparus* (adult/L4)	35 d
	0.5 mg/kg pour-on	*D viviparus* (adult/L4)	45 d
Ivermectin	0.2 mg/kg SC	*D viviparus* (adult/L4)	35 d
	0.5 mg/kg pour-on	*D viviparus* (adult/L4)	48 d
	0.2 mg/kg PO	*D filaria* (adult and L4)	11 d

Abbreviations: IM, intramuscularly; L4, Fourth-stage larvae; SC, subcutaneously.
[a] Follow current manufacturer's recommendations.
[b] Withdrawal times vary among the formulations.

practices such as grazing susceptible animals away from infected animals or moist, heavily contaminated pastures will limit the transmission of lungworm infection. A vaccine based on irradiated third-stage *D viviparus* larvae is commercially available in the United Kingdom and parts of western Europe; however, it is not available in the United States.

Dictyocaulus filaria

The life cycle of *D filaria* is similar to that of *D viviparus*. Adults live in the bronchi and trachea of goats and sheep. Embryonated eggs (112 to 135 μm by 52 to 67 μm) are coughed up, swallowed, and hatch in the small intestine [9,25]. First-stage larvae are passed to the environment in host feces, and, in the environment, larvae undergo two molts to the infective third stage. The rate of development of the larvae to third stage depends on humidity and temperature; however, this development can be achieved in less than a week. Infective larvae actively move from feces to herbage, remain near the soil, and are inadvertently ingested by the grazing host. Larvae exsheath in the small intestine, penetrate the intestinal wall within 18 hours of infection, and enter the right colic mesenteric lymph nodes, where they remain for 6 days, molting twice to fourth- and fifth-stage larvae. After day 7 post infection, they migrate via the thoracic duct to the anterior vena cava, heart, and pulmonary arteries. Larvae are in the lung tissue from day 8 to day 14, but after day 12 parasites move to the respiratory passages [26,27]. They penetrate the walls of the alveoli and enter the bronchioles and the bronchi, where they either arrest development or become sexually mature adults at about 4 weeks after infection. First-stage larvae may be seen in the feces at approximately 26 days after infection [25], with peak larval output occurring 39 to 57 days after infection [28].

D filaria is more prevalent in moist climates. Larvae survive for 2 to 3 months at moderate temperatures but are susceptible to desiccation. The ensheathed infective third-stage larvae are more resistant to desiccation than first- and second-stage larvae. Larvae are also resistant to the cold, with first- and second-stage larvae withstanding freezing temperatures for as long as 12 days and third-stage larvae surviving for as long as 19 days [25]. Consequently, larvae can survive on pasture throughout the winter. Spring pastures contaminated with larvae from the previous year and with larvae from adults developing from arrested larvae in ewes or yearlings are sources of infection for young, susceptible animals [29]. Acquisition of larvae can result in disease in lambs or kids during the second half of their first grazing season. Because both sheep and goats develop strong immunity to reinfection [30], disease is more common in young animals. This resistance to reinfection can last for as long as 46 months in sheep; however, its strength and duration appear to depend on the level and number of exposures and on the length of time before reinfection. Interestingly, *D filaria* can establish in the lungs of calves; although these do not result in patent infections, they have resulted in disease. Additionally, a degree of immunity is produced against subsequent challenge with *D viviparus* larvae [31].

Individual susceptibility to infection with *D filaria* varies; however, goats are more susceptible to infection and may be more severely affected than sheep [30]. Heavy infections can produce distinct clinical signs in both host species. Coughing develops 2 to 3 weeks after infection, when adult worms are maturing in the bronchi and trachea. Other signs include shallow, rapid breathing, lung rales, bilateral nasal discharge, loss of appetite, and loss of weight [25,28]. Death is uncommon. Bronchitis, pulmonary edema, collapse of lung tissue, and emphysema may occur [25,32]. Inflammatory reactions develop as larvae migrate into the alveoli, and macrophages, plasma cells, giant cells, leucocytes, and eosinophils invade the area. Larval migration into the bronchioles and bronchi and subsequent maturation to adults result in bronchitis characterized by the proliferation of bronchiolar epithelium and infiltration by leucocytes and eosinophils [25,32]. Aspiration of eggs and larvae into the bronchioles and alveoli may result in pneumonia. Atelectasis may occur when bronchi are blocked by parasites and mucus. Complications include secondary bacterial infections, which may result in bacterial pneumonia.

Parasitic bronchitis in sheep may be successfully treated with anthelmintics; however, strategic applications must be designed relative to the local epidemiology of the parasite. Formulations of albendazole, levamisole, and ivermectin are effective and labeled for the control of *D filaria* in sheep in the United States (see Table 1). Additionally, moxidectin (1% injectable; 0.2% oral drench; at 0.2 mg/kg) and doramectin (0.2 mg/kg intramuscularly) have been shown to be effective in sheep [33–35]. No products are currently labeled for the control of this parasite in goats; however, levamisole (7.5 mg/kg orally, subcutaneously), fenbendazole (5 to 10 mg/kg), and ivermectin (0.2 mg/kg) are reported to be effective [36]. Treatment interferes with the development of immunity in goats, so animals should not be returned to contaminated pastures. Management measures include the provision of dry pastures to reduce the development and survival of free-living larval stages. The majority of *D filaria* larvae are produced by relatively few animals [37]; therefore, treating or culling these animals may markedly reduce pasture contamination. Older animals, which may be clinically immune but capable of shedding first-stage larvae, should be grazed separately from susceptible kids and lambs.

Muellerius capillaris

The life cycle of *M capillaris* is indirect. Adults in the lung parenchyma of sheep and goats produce unsegmented eggs measuring 100 by 20 μm [9], which hatch in the lungs. First-stage larvae are released and move by way of the trachea to the intestine, where they pass with fecal material into the environment. First-stage larvae are resistant to desiccation and freezing temperatures and must invade a susceptible land mollusc to develop further [38]. Within the mollusc, larvae undergo two molts to the infective third stage. The rate of development to third stage depends on which of the many susceptible species of snails and slugs is infected. Sheep and goats become infected by inadvertently ingesting molluscs that contain infective third-stage larvae. Larvae are released from the snail during digestion, penetrate the intestinal wall, enter the mesenteric lymph nodes, and migrate via the thoracic duct to the heart, pulmonary arteries, and lung. Early fourth-stage larvae, fourth-stage larvae, and adults are found in nodules in the lung tissue. On occasion, nodules will degenerate and adults may be found in the bronchioles. Adults are present 25 to 38 days after infection and may survive and shed larvae for as long as 4.5 years [39]. Arrested development of larvae may prolong the prepatent period by approximately 5 to 6 weeks [25,40].

The longevity of adult parasites provides for prolonged contamination of pastures with first-stage larvae. Year-round shedding of larvae has been demonstrated in Ontario, Canada, in Maryland, United States, and in Britain [6,39,41]. Transmission to the definitive host depends on the survivability of these larvae on pasture and on the presence of an appropriate intermediate host. The ability of the parasite to survive for the lifetime of the mollusc and remain viable for a short time after its death further enhances its availability to grazing animals. In addition to the availability of intermediate hosts, prevalence is influenced by season, age of dairy goats, and the accumulation of larval stages in the lung [41]. Prevalences of 64% and 68% have been reported in dairy goats in Maryland [6] and Georgia [7], respectively.

Infection with *M capillaris* is generally not associated with clinical disease; however, impaired pulmonary gas exchange, reduced weights and breeding performance, and increased mortality have been reported in infected animals [39,42,43]. Infection is more pathogenic in goats, where low fecal larval counts may be associated with respiratory signs [4,40]. Heavy infections can result in interstitial pneumonia, broncho-pneumonia, or fibrinous pleuritis [9,44]. In sheep, distinct lung lesions appear as grayish subpleural nodules that range from less than 1 mm to several centimeters in diameter and are generally on the dorsal aspect of the diaphragmatic lobes [25,32,45]. Larger nodules are noncalcified brood capsules containing mature reproducing adults and first-stage larvae, whereas the smaller nodules contain remnants of immature or adult parasites and may be calcified. Numbers of brood capsules increase with the age of the host.

Although infections with *M capillaris* typically result in nodular lesions, a more diffuse lesion may also occur [44–46]. Infection may result in diffuse thickening of the alveolar septa, with mononuclear cell infiltrates and prominant fibromuscular hyperplasia. Both nodular and lobular lesions were observed in goats that had primary and secondary infections with *M capillaris* [46]. Mild cellular reactions were observed during primary infections; leucophilia in the bronchoalveolar spaces was present at 2 weeks post infection, when parasites were first established in lung tissue, and again at 7 to 9 weeks when numerous eggs were produced. Tissue reactions in secondary infections were more severe; macrophages, lymphocytes, and eosinophils infiltrated the lung tissue, type II cell hyperplasia occurred, and granulomas formed around the parasites [32,40,45,46]. Immunity was demonstrated in secondary infections by a longer prepatent period, reduced numbers of adult *Muellerius*, and reduced numbers of larvae shed in the feces [46]. However, older animals may have greater numbers of lungworm [39,41,47,48]. Secondary bacterial pneumonia may occur in subclinical *M capillaris* infections [44,47].

M capillaris infections are often inapparent and go untreated. No anthelmintics are labeled for this parasite in the United States; however, several are effective at reducing the number of first-stage larvae shed in feces (Table 2). Repeated anthelmintic treatment may be necessary, because shedding of larvae in feces resumes even in animals housed to prevent reinfection. Anthelmintics may be more effective against adults and less effective against inhibited larval stages. Larvae surviving treatment resume development, mature, and produce new first-stage larvae. Alternatively, anthelmintics may not eliminate all adults but may reduce their fecundity, resulting in a transient decrease in shedding of larvae [5,47,49]. Anthelmintic treatment and prevention of contact with the intermediate host through the provision

Table 2
Anthelmintics used for treatment and control of *Muellerius capillaris*

Drug[a]	Dosage	Host	Reference
Fenbendazole	30 mg/kg PO	Goats	[47,52]
	2 × 15 mg/kg PO 48 h apart	Goats	[5]
	1.25–5.0 mg/kg PO daily for 1–2 wk	Goats	[49]
	3 × 450 mg at 48-h intervals	Goats	[53]
Albendazole	1.0 mg/kg daily for 2 wk	Goats	[49]
Ivermectin	0.2 mg/kg PO	Goats	[47]
	0.2–0.3 mg/kg SC	Goats	[5,41]
Moxidectin	0.2 mg/kg SC; PO	Sheep	[54]

Abbreviation: SC, subcutaneously.
[a] Available in the United States.

of well-drained pasture and mollusc-free housing will limit infection with this parasite.

Diagnosis of lungworm infection

Antemortem diagnosis of lungworm infection depends on the recognition of clinical signs and knowledge of local parasite epidemiology and grazing history. Infection may be confirmed by the demonstration of first-stage larvae in fresh fecal material or of nematodes at necropsy. First-stage larvae are recovered from feces using the Baermann technique [50,51]. Recovered larvae may be identified to species by morphology [9]. First-stage *D viviparus* larvae measure 310 to 360 μm by 16 to 19 μm and have pointed tails and characteristic intestinal food granules. Infection in the pre- and postpatent phases of the disease, when larvae are not shed in feces, may be confirmed by the detection of immature stages in tracheal washes. Tracheal washes may also provide cytologic evidence of eosinophilic inflammation typical of parasitic bronchitis or pneumonia. First-stage *D filaria* larvae measure 500 to 540 μm by 25 μm and have a blunt tail and a small knob at their anterior end. Like *D viviparus,* these larvae have characteristic food granules in their intestinal cells. First-stage larvae of *M capillaris* measure 300 to 320 μm by 14 to 15 μm and have an undulating tail with a small dorsal spine at its base.

Postmortem diagnosis may be made by the identification of lungworms [9] and characteristic lung pathology at necropsy. Adult *D viviparus,* found in the bronchi and trachea, are long, thin white worms with small buccal cavities. Males are 17 to 50 mm in length and females are 23 to 80 mm. Adult *D filaria* may also be recovered from the bronchi and trachea at necropsy. Adult males are 25 to 80 mm long and have a short bursa, and adult females are 43 to 112 mm long with a conical, tapered tail. Adult *M capillaris* are found in the lung parenchyma. Males measure 11 to 14 mm by 32 to 35 μm and have a posterior end coiled in 11 to 13 spirals. Adult females are

19 to 23 mm by 40 to 50 μm. Eggs (100 by 20 μm) and larvae may be visible in tissue sections.

References

[1] Bliss DH, Myers GH. Lungworm (*Dictyocaulus*) outbreak in lactating dairy cows. Large Anim Pract 1998;19(2):20–3.
[2] Barling K, Wikse S, Field R, et al. An outbreak of lungworms in lightweight stocker calves. Compendium on Continuing Education for the Practicing Veterinarian 1998;20(Suppl 4): S104–9.
[3] Eddi CS, Williams JC, Swalley RA. Epidemiology of *Dictyocaulus viviparus* in Louisiana (U.S.A.). Vet Parasitol 1989;31(1):37–48.
[4] Lloyd S, Soulsby EJL. Survey of parasites in dairy goats. Am J Vet Res 1978;39(6):1057–9.
[5] McCraw BM, Menzies PI. Treatment of goats infected with the lungworm *Muellerius capillaris*. Can Vet J 1986;27(8):287–90.
[6] Ashraf M, Nepote KH. Prevalence of gastrointestinal nematodes, coccidia and lungworms in Maryland dairy goats. Small Rumin Res 1990;3(3):291–8.
[7] Anderson DL, Roberson EL. Gastrointestinal and respiratory parasitism in Georgia goats. Agri-Practice 1996;17(9):20–4.
[8] Mansfield LS, Gamble HR, Baker JS, et al. Lungworm infection in a sheep flock in Maryland. J Am Vet Med Assoc 1993;202(4):601–6.
[9] Levine ND. Lungworms and related nematodes. In: Nematode parasites of domestic animals and man. 2nd edition. Minneapolis (MN): Burgess Publishing Co.; 1980. p. 222–95.
[10] Jarrett WFH, McIntyre WIM, Urquhart GM. The pathology of experimental bovine parasitic bronchitis. J Pathol Bacteriol 1957;73(1):183–93.
[11] Soulsby EJL. Nematodes. In: Helminths, arthropods, and protozoa of domesticated animals. 7th edition. London: Lea & Febiger; 1982. p. 262–9.
[12] Jørgensen RJ. Spread of infective *Dictyocaulus viviparus* larvae in pasture and to grazing cattle: experimental evidence of the role of *Pilobolus* fungi. Vet Parasitol 1982;10(4):331–9.
[13] Lyons ET, Hemken RD, Button FS. Overwintering of larvae of the cattle lungworm (*Dictyocaulus viviparus*) on pasture in Kentucky. J Am Vet Med Assoc 1981;179(5):456–7.
[14] Winters JB, Worley DE. Distribution and seasonal prevalence of bovine lungworm in selected areas in western Montana. Am J Vet Res 1975;36:327–9.
[15] Jarrett WFH, McIntyre WI, Jennings FW, et al. The natural history of parasitic bronchitis with notes on prophylaxis and treatment. Vet Rec 1957;69:1329–36.
[16] Breeze R. Parasitic bronchitis and pneumonia. Vet Clin North Am Food Anim Pract 1985; 1(2):277–87.
[17] Poynter D. Parasitic bronchitis. In: Dawes B, editor. Advances in parasitology, Vol. 6. London and New York: Academic Press; 1968. p. 349–59.
[18] Ranjan S, DeLay R. Therapeutic and persistent efficacy of moxidectin 1% nonaqueous injectable formulation against natural and experimentally induced lung and gastrointestinal nematodes in cattle. Vet Parasitol 2004;120(4):305–17.
[19] Yazwinski TA, Williams JC, Smith LL, et al. Dose determination of the persistent activity of moxidectin long-acting injectable formulations against various nematode species in cattle. Vet Parasitol 2006;137(3–4):273–85.
[20] Downey NE. Effect of treatment with levamisole or fenbendazole on primary experimental *Dictyocaulus viviparus* infection and on resistance in calves. Vet Rec 1980;107(12):271–5.
[21] Borgsteede FH, de Leeuw WA, vd Burg WP. A comparison of the efficacy of four different long-acting boluses to prevent infections with *Dictyocaulus viviparus* in calves. Vet Q 1988; 10(3):177–86.
[22] Höglund J, Gånheim C, Alenius S. The effect of treatment with eprinomectin on lungworms at early patency on the development of immunity in young cattle. Vet Parasitol 2003;114(3): 205–14.

[23] Taylor SM, Kenny J, Edgar HW, et al. Induction of protective immunity to *Dictyocaulus viviparus* in calves while under treatment with endectocides. Vet Parasitol 2000;88(3–4): 219–28.
[24] Ploeger HW. *Dictyocaulus viviparus*: re-emerging or never been away? Trends Parasitol 2002; 18(8):329–32.
[25] Rose JH. Lungworms of the domestic pig and sheep. In: Dawes B, editor. Advances in parasitology, Vol. 11. London and New York: Academic Press; 1973. p. 559–99.
[26] Anderson PJS, Verster A. Studies on *Dictyocaulus filaria* II. Migration of the developmental stages in lambs. Onderstepoort J Vet Res 1971;38(3):185–90.
[27] Verster A, Collins HM, Anderson PJS. Studies on *Dictyocaulus filaria* IV. The morphogenesis of the parasitic stages in lambs. Onderstepoort J Vet Res 1971;38(3):199–206.
[28] Goldberg A. Experimental infection of sheep and goats with the nematode lungworm Dictyocaulus filaria. Am J Vet Res 1952;13(49):531–6.
[29] Ayalew L, Frechette JL, Malo R, et al. Seasonal fluctuation and inhibited development of populations of *Dictyocaulus filaria* in ewes and lambs. Can J Comp Med 1974;38(4): 448–56.
[30] Wilson GI. The strength and duration of immunity to *Dictyocaulus filaria* infection in sheep and goats. Res Vet Sci 1970;11(1):7–17.
[31] Parfitt JW, Sinclair IJ. Cross resistance to *Dictyocaulus viviparus* produced by *Dictyocaulus filaria* infections in calves. Res Vet Sci 1967;8(6):6–13.
[32] Poynter D. Some tissue reactions to the nematode parasites of animals. In: Dawes B, editor. Advances in parasitology, Vol. 4. London and New York: Academic Press; 1966. p. 321–83.
[33] Dorchies P, Cardinaud B, Fournier R. Efficacy of moxidectin as a 1% injectable solution and a 0.1% oral drench against nasal bots, pulmonary and gastrointestinal nematodes in sheep. Vet Parasitol 1996;65(1–2):163–8.
[34] Gicik Y, Arslan MÖ, Sari B. Efficacy of doramectin against gastrointestinal nematodes and lungworms in naturally infected pregnant sheep. Turkish Journal of Veterinary and Animal Sciences 2002;26:793–7.
[35] Hidalgo-Argüello MR, Díez-Baños N, Rojo-Vázquez FA. Efficacy of moxidectin 1% injectable and 0.2% oral drench against natural infection by *Dictyocaulus filaria* in sheep. Vet Parasitol 2002;107(1–2):95–101.
[36] Smith MC, Sherman DM. Respiratory system. In: Goat medicine. Malvern (PA): Lea & Febiger; 1994. p. 247–74.
[37] Sreter T, Molnar V, Kassai T. The distribution of nematode egg counts and larval counts in grazing sheep and their implications for parasite control. Int J Parasitol 1994;24(1): 103–8.
[38] Solomon A, Ilan P, Itamar G. Desiccation tolerance of *Muellerius* cf. *capillaris* (Nematoda: Protostrongylidae) first-stage larvae. J Parasitol 1998;84(4):802–5.
[39] Rose JH. Some observations on the transmission of lungworm infection in a flock of sheep at pasture. Res Vet Sci 1965;6:189–95.
[40] Sauerländer R. Experimental infection of sheep and goats with *Muellerius capillaris* (Protostrongylidae, Nematoda). J Vet Med B Infect Dis Vet Public Health 1988;35:525–48.
[41] McCraw BM, Menzies PI. *Muellerius capillaris*: resumption of shedding larvae in feces following anthelmintic treatment and prevalence in housed goats. Can Vet J 1988;29(5): 453–4.
[42] Berrag B, Cabaret J. Impaired pulmonary gas exchange in ewes naturally infected by small lungworms. Int J Parasitol 1996;26(12):1397–400.
[43] Berrag B, Cabaret J. Gastrointestinal and pulmonary nematode infections decrease goat productivity in Moroccan semi-arid conditions. J Helminthol 1998;72(1):15–20.
[44] Nimmo JS. Six cases of verminous pneumonia (*Muellerius* sp.) in goats. Can Vet J 1979; 20(2):49–52.
[45] Beresford-Jones WP. Observations on *Muellerius capillaris* (Müller, 1889) Cameron, 1927 III. Experimental infection of sheep. Res Vet Sci 1967;8:272–9.

[46] Berrag B, Rhalem A, Sahibi H, et al. Bronchoalveolar cellular responses of goats following infections with *Muellerius capillaris* (Protostrongylidae, Nematoda). Vet Immunol Immunopathol 1997;58(1):77–88.
[47] Gregory E, Foreyt WJ, Breeze R. Efficacy of ivermectin and fenbendazole against lungworms. Vet Med 1985;80(2):114–7.
[48] Polley L. Quantitative observations on intrapulmonary populations of *Muellerius capillaris* (Mueller, 1889) Cameron, 1927, in sheep. J Parasitol 1987;73(1):234–6.
[49] Helle O. The efficacy of fenbendazole and albendazole against the lungworm *Muellerius capillaris* in goats. Vet Parasitol 1986;22(3–4):293–301.
[50] Eysker M. The sensitivity of the Baermann method for the diagnosis of primary *Dictyocaulus viviparus* infections in calves. Vet Parasitol 1997;69(1–2):89–93.
[51] McKenna PB. Comparative evaluation of two emigration/sedimentation techniques for the recovery of dictyocaulid and protostrongylid larvae from faeces. Vet Parasitol 1999;80(4): 345–51.
[52] Bliss EL, Greiner EC. Efficacy of fenbendazole and cambendazole against *Muellerius capillaris* in dairy goats. Am J Vet Res 1985;46(9):1923–5.
[53] McCraw BM, Eaton EW, Ogilvie TH, et al. Transmission and treatment of *Muellerius capillaris* in goats. Can Vet J 1981;22(6):205.
[54] Papadopoulos E, Sotiraki S, Himonas C, et al. Treatment of small lungworm infestation in sheep by using moxidectin. Vet Parasitol 2004;121(3–4):329–36.

ELSEVIER
SAUNDERS

Vet Clin Food Anim
22 (2006) 595–611

VETERINARY
CLINICS
Food Animal Practice

Tritrichomonas foetus

D. Owen Rae, DVM, MPVM[a,*],
John E. Crews, DVM, MS[b]

[a]*Food Animal Reproduction and Medicine Service, Veterinary Medical Center, College of Veterinary Medicine, University of Florida, PO Box 100136, Gainesville, FL 32610-0136, USA*
[b]*Florida Department of Agriculture and Consumer Services, State of Florida, 6470 Lake Buffum Road South, Fort Meade, FL 33841, USA*

Historical overview

The disease caused by *Tritrichomonas foetus* was originally described by Kunstler in 1888. Its discovery, however, is attributed to the Italian scientist Mazzanti in 1900. Mazzanti reported trichomonads in two cows and one heifer that were slaughtered because of infertility. Its discovery occurred in the same time frame as brucellosis (1897), which may have limited *T foetus* research. The next reported work on the disease occurred in Germany between 1924 and 1929 by Drescher, Riedmüller, and Abelein [1].

In 1928 Riedmüller documented the results of a study of 105 aborted fetuses with nine cases involving trichomonads. At this time the name of *Trichomonas foetus* was proposed [1].

The first reported case of trichomonosis in cattle in the United States occurred in 1932, when Emmerson [2] found trichomonads in the vaginas of two infertile cows. The diagnosis was made by microscopic examination of vaginal smears. The second case was reported in Iowa by McNutt, Walsh, and Murray [1]. Since 1933, the reports have been published from numerous sources from all over the world.

Taxonomic classification

Traditional classification schemes separating the Protozoa into four divisions and placing *T foetus* within the Sarcomastigophora have recently been abandoned in favor of a hierarchical approach without formal rank

* Corresponding author.
E-mail address: RaeO@mail.vetmed.ufl.edu (D.O. Rae).

doi:10.1016/j.cvfa.2006.07.001 ***vetfood.theclinics.com***

designations [3–5]. Using this scheme, the position of the organism referred to is followed by two or three higher ranks placed in brackets, with the highest rank first. Under this system, then, the organism referred to is *Tritrichomonas foetus* and should be written as *Tritrichomonas foetus* [Excavata: Parabasalia].

Structure

The trichomonads are pleomorphic but are generally pyriform-shaped protozoa with a rounded anterior end and generally a pointed posterior. *T foetus* is approximately 20 × 10 μm and has a single nucleus and four flagella. The flagella arise from the kinetosome complex at the anterior end. Three of the flagella are free anteriorly, whereas the fourth extends backward. An undulating membrane, with three to five waves and a characteristic vibrating movement, gives it a distinct diagnostic feature when comparing *T foetus* to most other protozoans found in preputial samples contaminated with fecal material.

Serotype and antigenic differentiation

Serotypes of *T foetus* have been described and were established using agglutination, passive hemagglutination, and skin tests [3,6]. More commonly, three serotypes, identified as var. *brisbane*, var. *belfast*, and var. *manley*, have been described. The conclusion is that antigenic types appear to have no important role in the immunity of *T foetus* because heifers immunized with one serotype develop resistance to infections from homologous and heterologous strains [3].

Hall and colleagues [7] reported that the *T foetus* antigens were a highly complex set of 55 to 60 protein bands with molecular weights ranging from approximately 25 kD to greater than 210 to 220 kD. Of these, 38 were identified as probable antigens in the same molecular weight range. The similarity of the total protein profiles among *T foetus* isolates and the similarity in antigen profiles revealed by antiserum indicate strong antigenic cross-reactions among diverse isolates of *T foetus* [8].

Problematic taxonomic differentiation of *T foetus* and *T suis*

A subject of controversy also exists in the synonymy of *T foetus* and *T suis* (in swine). This synonymy stimulates problematic issues with the pathogenicity and life cycle of *T foetus*. Several investigators have reported that trichomonad cultures from swine (nasal and digestive tracts) when inoculated into the reproductive tracts of cattle caused apparent infections [9,10]. Fitzgerald's study [10] indicated that natural infections of the bovine genital tract with porcine trichomonads may occur when pigs and cows are kept in the same or adjacent areas. This controversy continued, based on the lack of differences in structure and cultivation of *T foetus* and *T suis* [11]. Recently the random amplified polymorphic DNA technique was used to comparatively assess several isolates of *T foetus*, *T suis*, and *T mobilensis* (in squirrel monkeys [12]). This study indicated that all *T foetus* and *T suis* isolates resulted in identical genomic fingerprints, which would additionally support genetic identity between the two trichomonads. Felleisen and colleagues [12] further suggested those trichomonads from cattle and swine represent variants of the same species that vary primarily in differences in possible pathogenicity and host range. Although the synonymy is accepted by many, this issue has not yet been resolved and warrants further microbiologic and epidemiologic studies.

Pathogenesis

In the male

Venereal diseases of most domestic animals have one thing in common. In the male, the effects of the disease are limited to that of an asymptomatic carrier, whereas the negative clinical effects of infection occur in the female. *T foetus* localizes in the secretions of the epithelial lining of the penis, prepuce, and distal urethra. Microscopically, the organism does not invade the epithelium. There are no observable changes in semen quality attributable to the organism's presence [13,14]. This feature does not, however, preclude the contamination of the semen from a preputial source [15]. There is rarely more than a scant purulent discharge from the prepuce during the first two weeks of an infection, which never develops into significant pathologic lesions [16].

The most important feature of *T foetus* infection in the bull is development of the chronic carrier state. This phenomenon is believed to be related to deepening of the epithelial crypts of the penis and prepuce as the bull ages (age 3–4 years and older). The assumption is that deepening of the crypts provides a more suitable microaerophilic environment, which supports establishment of the chronic infection [17]. It is generally assumed that young bulls (less than 3 years of age) are transient carriers and remain infected for only brief periods. Clark and coworkers [18] established experimental *T foetus* infections in 12 of 13 bulls of ages 3 to 7 years compared with 3 of 19 that were 1 to 2 years of age. Studies suggest that reduction in the incidence of infection can be achieved by using young bulls alone. Christensen and colleagues [19] examined a herd of 300 Shorthorn and Santa Gertrudis bulls (8 years old) that were removed from the herd and replaced with 325 young Brahman bulls (2 years old). Before introduction of the replacement bulls, 47% of bulls were found to be culture positive. After 1 year, a sampling of the replacement bulls (99 bulls) revealed a 1% prevalence of *T foetus*. At 2 years, 80 bulls were sampled and the prevalence had increased to

4%. At 4 years postintroduction (6 years of age), 112 of the bulls were slaughtered and samples of the prepuce and penis revealed 15 of the 112 were culture positive (13.4% prevalence) [20]. The precipitous rise was correlated to the increasing age of bulls. Age alone does not preclude the possibility of the carrier state existing, however, even in bulls as young as 2 years of age [21].

Breed susceptibility has been examined as a risk factor also. BonDurant and coworkers [22] showed a greater prevalence among *Bos taurus* bulls than bulls of *B indicus* origin. There was, however, no biologic significance attributed to this variation because of a lack of equal distribution of breeds across all herds. Rae and colleagues [23] evaluated breed susceptibility in a large multiple breed cow–calf enterprise. They found the highest prevalence of *T foetus* in Brangus bulls (17.9%) and the lowest prevalence in Braford bulls (2.5%), both of which are *B taurus* × *B indicus* breeds. In that study, the prevalence in Angus bulls (*B taurus*, the only *B taurus* breed represented) was 12%, being within the middle range of other bull groups. Further, in a study reported by Rae and colleagues [24], *B taurus* bulls were six times more likely to be culture positive than *B indicus* bulls. Within the *B taurus* group, several breeds were more likely to be culture positive for *T foetus*, namely, Simmental, Charolais, and Angus. Although several studies have examined breed predilections, none have been able to establish a clear breed association for bull susceptibility to trichomonosis [22,24,25].

The venereal transmission of *T foetus* occurs when an infected bull breeds a susceptible female (cow or heifer) or a susceptible bull breeds an infected female. Clark and coworkers [26] performed experiments to ascertain if transmission could occur through passive methods (ie, a noninfected bull transferring the organism to an uninfected female after a mating to a known infected female). In the experiments, topical application of 2×10^6 *T foetus* organisms to the external vulva failed to cause infection, whereas deposition of similar number of organisms to the anterior vagina caused all animals to become infected. Furthermore, experiments with this group of artificially infected cows (10) and 15 nonexposed cows led to 2 of 15 (13%) becoming infected as a result of service following a breeding with the known infected female. The estimated time interval required for the passive transmission of infection was less than 20 minutes. Compared with the breeding by a known infected bull to a susceptible cow, the passive transmission of the organism by uninfected bulls to unexposed cows following breeding of an infected cow is much less important in the transmission of this disease. Using young bulls in an infected herd thus does not eliminate the risk for disease transfer, but can be used to moderate the overall transmission effect.

T foetus infection also has been associated with bull factors related to herd and herd management practices. Rae and colleagues [24] reported that the likelihood of disease was greatest in larger herds under more extensive management settings (ie, 500 or greater cows/herd, 53.9% prevalence, compared with medium-sized herds of 100 to 499 cows, 10% prevalence).

Herd management practices that increased the bull-to-cow ratio or increased the number of bulls per breeding group (where there were large herd numbers often on large tracts) also increased the likelihood of disease. These factors are believed to have increased the number of sexual contacts by infected bulls and thus amplified the likelihood of disease.

In the female

T foetus gains entry through coital exposure from a persistently infected male or passive transfer from a previously uninfected bull that has had recent coitus with an infected female. Subsequently, a mild vaginitis may occur that may go undetected. The organism gains entry into the uterine lumen via the cervix during estrus [27]. Colonization of the entire reproductive tract with *T foetus* occurs within 1 to 2 weeks.

The infection that results may interfere with fertilization and development of the resultant embryo [28]. If the conceptus dies, it most commonly occurs by 50 to 70 days of gestation [29]. Death of the embryo or fetus during this early stage of pregnancy results in a prolonged interestrous interval [27].

Clearance of the *T foetus* organism from the female is quite variable. In heifers, the duration of infection is reported to be as short as 95 days [29] or as long as 22 months [30]. Skirrow and BonDurant [31] detected organisms in the reproductive tract for 13 to 28 weeks after experimental infection in heifers.

Clark and colleagues [28] reported a more adverse effect on calving interval during the first and second year of a herd infection. Their data suggested that cows infected with *T foetus* had an increase in the calving interval of 96 and 98 days respectively during the first two years of infection when compared with cows mated to noninfected bulls.

Clark and coworkers [28] also reported that cows exposed to *T foetus* did not develop long-term immunity to reinfection and suggested that the susceptibility to secondary and tertiary infections was directly related to the elapsed time from the previous infection. They estimated that the convalescent immunity did not persist beyond 15 months. This scenario follows the more common condition when cows become infected and expel or reabsorb the embryo while it is still small in mass.

Pyometra and abortion are the first physical signs of a *T foetus* infection in a herd, but are believed to occur in less than 5% of infected cows [32]. Pyometra results as the corpus luteum of pregnancy is maintained, followed by a large purulent response. By the time pyometra is detected, the uterine mucosa may have suffered damage [3].

The existence of a persistent infection in females has been documented by Skirrow [33]. This persistence is defined as any female that carries the infection through a gestation and into the subsequent breeding season. These cows provide a source of continued infection in the herd. Although this is estimated to occur infrequently (<1%), this potential source of infection emphasizes that control programs must focus on the entire herd, not just the bull.

Rhyan and coworkers [34] reported pathologic changes in several late-term *T foetus* aborted fetuses. One third of the *T foetus* abortions occurred in the last trimester. There were consistent patterns of placental and fetal lesions that were attributable to *T foetus*. All placentas examined had focal or diffuse invasion of the chorionic stroma by *T foetus*. The organisms were clearly discernible on hematoxylin and eosin (HE)–stained sections of non-autolyzed placentas. The characteristic flagella and undulating membrane were not discernible on the HE-stained sections, but Bodian's silver protargol stain best demonstrated these features. In some of the placentas there was evidence of a moderate inflammatory cell infiltrate composed predominately of mononuclear cells. The epithelium of the placenta and its adherent necrotic debris were examined, but were rarely discernible. Six of the 11 fetuses examined had bronchopneumonia with identifiable trichomonads in airways. Four of the cases had phagocytized organisms in the cytoplasm of the macrophages. Two of the fetuses had a marked interstitial pneumonia. Trichomonads were also identified in sections of esophagus, abomasum, and intestine. One fetus examined had focal coagulative necrosis of the centrilobular hepatocytes. These findings, lesions in the fetus and the placenta of late-term abortions, support the observed occurrence of persistently infected females, "carrier cows".

Rhyan and colleagues [35] further described a tissue-invasive effect in four third-trimester abortions attributable to *T foetus*. Microscopic lesions were similar in all fetuses. In particular, necrotizing enteritis and pyogranulomatous bronchopneumonia with tissue invasion by trichomonads was evident. The mechanism that produced the mucosal injury was not determined.

The exact mechanism that leads to the death of the conceptus is not known. Burgess and coworkers [36] described cytotoxic and hemolytic effects by *T foetus* on mammalian cells. Burgess and McDonald [37] found a surface adhesin (190,000 molecular weight) that has an important role in *T foetus* adhering to mammalian cells. A similar adhesin and cytologic effect has been described with a venereal trichomonad of humans, *Trichomonas vaginalis* [38]. Identification of the surface adhesin is just one step in understanding the mechanism that leads to pregnancy wastage that occurs in trichomonosis.

Aydintug and colleagues [39] investigated the interactions between *T foetus* and host defenses in the bovine reproductive tract to determine the role of classic and alternative pathways of bovine complement in killing of this organism. They reported that *T foetus* was susceptible to killing by bovine complement. The presence of specific antibody greatly enhanced complement-mediated killing. Their study suggests that the surface of *T foetus* is capable of activating the alternative pathway of bovine complement, which implies that antibody and complement can promote protection against *T foetus*.

Aydintug and coworkers [40] also evaluated the role of the leukocyte in the killing of *T foetus* by specific bovine antibody and complement. They found that neutrophils alone were only slightly effective in killing *T foetus*.

Also, addition of specific antibody alone did not enhance the bovine neutrophil–mediated killing. When trichomonads were first opsonized with antibody and complement combined, then maximal killing of *T foetus* occurred when exposed to bovine neutrophils.

Impact on production as a result of the pathology

The primary impact of this disease is the elongation of the calving interval (days between consecutive calvings). Elongation of the calving interval decreases the average number of days to target weaning dates. This delay in obtaining optimal marketable weights either forces calves to be marketed at lighter weight or increases feeding cost to reach a desired market weight. Either scenario reduces herd performance and profitability. The effects were estimated by Rae [41] using a simulation model of the disease and indicated that a reduction in annual calf crop of 14% to 50% could occur if bull infection prevalence increased from 20% to 40%. The disease thus has staggering consequences worldwide [42–44].

Diagnosis of *Tritrichomonas foetus*

T foetus infections in cattle present a diagnostic challenge for the cattle industry. The disease may go undetected in a herd because of its insidious nature. The features of disease expression characteristic of trichomonosis (the nonclinical carrier state of bulls, the occasional overt signs of infertility in females, and the eventual conception with the mere lengthening of the calving interval in infected females) are not pathognomonic signs of the disease. These same distinguishing features are expressed in other infectious diseases (ie, *Campylobacter foetus*, *Leptospira hardjo*, and *Ureaplasm* sp, and various nutritional conditions [17,45]. For this reason diagnostic testing must be used to diagnose trichomonosis. A positive diagnosis of *T foetus* is by demonstration of the organism in either the living form by microscopic examination (with or without the use of in vitro culture systems) or detection of DNA markers by polymerase chain reaction (PCR) amplification systems. Attempts to develop a serologic test to detect the immunologic response resulting from exposure to *T foetus* have been unsuccessful or limited in their application [46].

Microscopic examination of *T foetus*

Microscopic examination of suspended preputial secretions, smegma, and fluids from the male, and cervicovaginal mucus or uterine fluid from the female, was the first routine method used in the diagnosis of trichomonosis [2]. Wet-mount microscopic samples are prepared by suspending a drop of smegma from the bull or fluid from the reproductive tract of the female on a microscopic slide. If the specimen is dry or too concentrated, it can be suspended in physiologic saline to improve the visibility. Evaluation may be done with or without the aid of a coverslip. Without a coverslip, a systematic evaluation of the slide must be done at all levels of the suspended drop. Use of a coverslip narrows the depth of field, helping in sample evaluation. The slide is examined for the presence of the *T foetus* organism at a ×100 magnification. Trichomonads display a characteristic spiral, jerky movement [4]. The diagnosis is made by the morphologic characteristics of *T foetus*. This diagnosis is done at ×400 magnification or greater to properly visualize the three anterior flagella, one posterior flagellum, and the undulating membrane. Several protozoal organisms resembling *T foetus* can be found as contaminants of the bovine reproductive tract. Relying on a diagnosis from characteristic movement without direct visualization of the morphologic features may result in an incorrect diagnosis [47–49].

Direct microscopic examinations of specimens for *T foetus* are diagnostic, but less sensitive than the use of in vitro culture systems [50–52]. There are several obvious reasons for this reduced sensitivity that relate to the environmental conditions commonplace to livestock-handling systems. In the authors' experience, rarely does one find the proper physical setting and time to perform direct microscopic examination of specimens adequately at the time of collection. Dust, wind, and direct sunlight are just a few of the conditions that increase the probability of an inaccurate diagnosis when relying on direct examination alone. Second, routine collections from bulls or females yield very small specimens that may have very low numbers of organisms. Sampling techniques can directly affect ability to recover and multiply the organism by culture, which is discussed later in this section.

Many culture and transport media systems have been described and most are generally effective growth media [4,53–55]. In the United States from mid-1940 until the late 1980s samples were most often obtained by preputial scraping and cultured on Diamond's medium [55]. In the early 1990s a proprietary medium that was marketed in a plastic pouch, *InPouch TF*, was introduced by BioMed (Biomed Diagnostics, Inc., San Jose, CA). Modified Diamond's medium [53,56] and *InPouch TF* have been compared and their relative sensitivity has been shown to be similar [55,57]. The *InPouch TF* has become the industry standard because of its availability and ease of use. The sensitivity (the proportion of true positives that are correctly identified by the test) of using culture media in the diagnosis of *T foetus* has been estimated at 81% to 95% [21,32,55]. After samples have been collected and placed in the media, they should be maintained at 37°C and protected from extremes in environmental conditions while being transported to the laboratory [57].

Samples should be maintained at 37°C during the laboratory evaluation period. Laboratory examination of cultures begins 24 to 48 hours after arrival at the laboratory. Samples are read at least every 48 hours for 5 to

7 days [53,58]. The modified Diamond's medium is examined either by direct microscopy from the bottom of the culture tube using an inverted microscope or by carefully aspirating 0.1 mL of the medium from the bottom of the medium and placing that fluid on a microscope slide. The *InPouch TF* samples are read using Biomed's special plastic microscope clip that holds the plastic pouch for microscopic evaluation. The Biomed system is designed to be evaluated without withdrawing medium from the plastic pouch. Both media systems are initially evaluated at ×100 magnification to scan the samples. The final morphologic determination should be made at ×400 magnification [47]. In vitro culture systems using modified Diamond's medium and Biomed's *InPouch TF* have been considered the gold standard and are efficient methods of *T foetus* diagnosis. Diagnostic methods based strictly on culture and morphology may lack in specificity (the proportion of true negatives that are correctly identified by the test), however, because of the presence of nonpathogenic trichomonad species in diagnostic specimens. PCR assays add a new level of confirmation and are discussed later.

Sampling techniques used in bulls and affect on diagnosis

Three methodologies—swab, douche, and pipette (scraping)—are described as sampling techniques to obtain specimens for diagnostic procedures. These have been used with various degrees of success in bulls. The first method, the cotton swab technique, is described by Morgan (1946) [1]. This procedure is effective for *Leptospira* sp when coupled with a transport media, but is rarely used for *T foetus* cultures in the United States.

The douche method is the preferred method of obtaining a culture sample in Europe [55]. Preference for preputial washing differs from Fitzgerald and colleagues [59] and Mikelsen [60], who indicate a preference for a dry collection method. Schönmann and coworkers [55] state, however, that the two diagnostic methods, dry pipette and douche method, are not statistically different.

The dry method is the preferred sampling technique in the United States. This scraping technique uses a sterile 18-in plastic insemination pipette that is introduced into the fornix and is scraped repeatedly and vigorously with and without suction applied by either a rubber bulb or a 12- to 20-mL disposable syringe. The scraping is vigorous and may cause the fluid to be slightly blood-tinged. The smegma may be directly placed in the culture media.

Sampling females and affect on diagnosis

Comparisons of diagnostic methods for detection of *T foetus* infections have been focused primarily on the bull. Isolation of organisms from the female is reported to be less sensitive when compared with the bull techniques [52,61]. Kittel and coworkers [62] indicated that the *InPouch TF* system was more effective than Diamond's medium (88% versus 68%) in detecting heifers that had been experimentally infected. The ability of the cow to eliminate an infection generally is recognized as requiring from 1 to 4 months [27]. Kittel and coworkers [62] suggested that the accuracy of prevalence studies in the cow depends on the timing of sampling relative to exposure. The immune response in females begins to eliminate the infection within 8 to 10 weeks after exposure in unvaccinated females [31]. For this reason, cultures from females are best performed before the infection is potentially eliminated by the immune response [62].

Sample handling and affect on diagnosis

There has been much discussion of sample handling and its affect on diagnosis. Skirrow and colleagues [21] discussed the time between *T foetus* collection and placement in an in vitro culturing medium. Placing specimens in a non-nutrient transport medium (eg, lactated Ringers) for transport to the laboratory then transferring to a culture medium reduced the sensitivity of diagnosis by up to 14%. With regard to temperature and media type, Bryan and coworkers [57] reported that when field or laboratory isolates were cultured in Diamond's medium or *InPouch TF*, all the cultures were positive when maintained for up to 4 days at either 22° or 37°C. This finding agreed with earlier work by Borchardt and colleagues [58] and Appell and colleagues [54]. Samples maintained at 4°C or less, however, resulted in inconsistent sensitivity (49% to 0%). Consequently, time, temperature, type of isolate, and type of media have an effect on the sensitivity of *T foetus* in vitro culture systems. It is therefore recommended that samples be placed on either Diamond's medium or *InPouch TF* immediately on collection and placed in an incubator that moderates the temperature between 22° to 37°C. Transport to the laboratory should be as expedient as prudent. These procedures are important in attaining diagnostic culture sensitivity for *T foetus*.

Polymerase chain reaction test for trichomonosis

The first PCR assay for diagnostic determination of trichomonosis in cattle was reported in 1991 [42,63]. Initial reports were promising, but subsequent field testing indicated that it lacked adequate sensitivity when compared with in vitro culture systems [54]. Assays using PCR amplification systems [64,65] continued in their development throughout the 1990s. Several issues were limiting the sensitivity of the various PCR assays, including DNA degradation, accumulation of inhibitory compounds, sample contamination, and unexpected amplification products, which could lead to inaccuracies in diagnosis [66]. Mukhufhi and colleagues [66] found that there was a decline in sensitivity of PCR testing with samples that were stored.

This decline was highly significant if the samples were stored 5 days or more. This loss of sensitivity with time was not prevented by the addition of the chaotropic agent guanidinium thiocyanate. In contrast, the results of the PCR were in 100% agreement with the culture as long as the PCR was performed within 24 hours of the sample being submitted.

The correct identification of nonpathogenic intestinal or coprophilic trichomonads (*Pentatrichomonas hominis*, *Tetratrichomonas* spp, and others) also continued to present a diagnostic challenge that had to be overcome for the PCR assays to be an effective diagnostic tool. Recently, several PCR assays have been described [67–71]. Campero and coworkers [68] described a two-step assay using culture followed by PCR confirmation of culture-positive samples to differentiate non-*T foetus* trichomonads. Grahn and coworkers [70] described a pan-trichomonad PCR assay that allows for the amplification of various trichomonad species. This single-step assay is able to discriminate between *T foetus* and various nonpathogenic intestinal trichomonads from various hosts. This assay's advantage is the elimination of false negatives that may result from failed amplification in a two-step PCR assay.

All of the recent PCR assays described above provide new useful tools in the correct identification of *T foetus*–infected bulls and identifying bulls that may have nonpathogenic trichomonads. Further field testing will validate the usefulness of these new assays. Until such time, a combination of in vitro culture methods and confirmation of the diagnostic status of the positive cultures with an appropriate PCR assay can provide a useful approach to diagnosis of this disease with quite acceptable diagnostic sensitivity and specificity.

Prevention and control of *Tritrichomonas foetus*

Richey [72] described four factors that outline the basic principles involved in any general disease-prevention program.

- Recognize the disease challenge (diagnosis and surveillance)
- Know when and why a challenge occurs (pathogenesis)
- Lower (or eradicate) the challenge (management)
- Raise the resistance to the specific disease challenge (immunology)

Previous sections of this document have described the first two principles, pathogenesis and diagnosis of *T foetus*. This section reviews the current prevention and control methodologies described for reducing challenge and increasing resistance to *T foetus* in beef cattle herds. Disease prevention is important to herds both with and without exposure to *T foetus*. A herd health program should prevent introduction of disease in a herd or reduce the exposure probability in affected herds. The measures discussed can be used to prevent the disease, lower the risk for disease, or eradicate trichomonosis from a herd.

Prevention of Tritrichomonas foetus *in beef herds*

Prevention of *T foetus* in a beef herd involves the application of basic cattle husbandry practices that are common principles for optimal animal health and productivity. Some elements of a prevention program that have been described to reduce the risk for introducing trichomonosis in a herd include:

- Control animal movement. This control includes good fencing. Preventing the entry of infected animals, both male and female, is an important front line to preventing *T foetus* in a herd [17].
- Avoid communal grazing of cattle on public lands. This practice is more common and of a greater concern in the western range regions of the United States [73].
- Purchase only virgin bulls or heifers as replacements. Because this disease is acquired through venereal contact, preferentially use animals that have had no known previous sexual contact. Use of virgin bulls less than 3 years of age also decreases the probability of a permanent carrier state. Young bulls decrease the number of infective sexual contacts within the herd, thus potentially decreasing the incidence of infection [14].
- Obtain preputial culture samples on all purchased bulls. This recommendation should also apply to unexposed bulls (virgin bulls). It has been said that "there is no such thing as a virgin bull" because the libido of young bulls predisposes them to sexual contact even if it is unplanned or unseen [17].
- Ideally, purchased cows and heifers should be bred separately, confirmed as pregnant, then pastured separately. To minimize risk for exposure from carrier cows, segregation should continue at least through the next breeding season [32].
- Keep the average age of herd bulls as young as possible. Increasing age is a risk factor for bulls to become permanent carriers of the disease [14,23].
- Use a limited length (60–90 days) breeding season. A long breeding season can mask productivity losses attributable to *T foetus* [74].
- Do not commingle cows or heifers of unknown status during a breeding season [32]. Use control methods, specifically immunization, for other diseases such as campylobacter and leptospirosis. These diseases are common and cause problems similar to trichomonosis [74].

Control of Tritrichomonas foetus *in beef herds*

Therapy for bulls infected with *T foetus* at one time involved treatment with nitroimidazole derivatives, such as dimetridazole, ipronidazole, and metronidazole [52,75,76]. Currently, however, there are no effective, approved medications for use in cattle in the United States. The extralabel use of the imidazole derivatives in food-producing animals is strictly forbidden [17].

When *T foetus* has been confirmed in a herd, following all of the above preventative measures provides important tools in the elimination of this disease. Some additional measures should be considered to accelerate an eradication program, however.

- Hasten testing and removal of infected bulls. This procedure should be done well before the breeding season. A single test, preputial culture, is reported to have an 85% probability of identifying a bull that is indeed culture positive. Three sequential tests at 1- to 2-week intervals have a 99% probability of identifying a bull infected with *T foetus* [52]. Further, the procedure of multiple testing of infected herd bulls should continue until no new cases are identified. Once successful control has been achieved, yearly screening can be performed at the time of breeding soundness examinations to monitor herd status.
- Purchase test-negative herd sires. Know the disease status of the herd where bulls are purchased and insist that bulls have a negative culture and a satisfactory breeding soundness evaluation.
- Reduce the average age of the bull herd. Use bulls of no more than 6 years of age. This limit may be considered an extreme measure, but reducing the overall bull age reduces the probability of permanent carriers. Carrier bulls prolong the problem in the herd.
- Single-sire herds lower the exposure potential to disease, but this is often impractical in large commercial operations. Large numbers of bulls in a breeding unit have been associated with greater economic loss [23].
- Breed the same bulls with the same cattle from breeding season to breeding season until the disease has been brought under control. Any changes of bulls within a breeding unit should be done only after assuring that they have had three negative cultures at weekly intervals.
- Reduce the breeding season length to no more than 90 to 120 days and perform a pregnancy examination 45 to 60 days thereafter. Open cows should be culled or placed in a high-risk herd to reduce spread to susceptible cows. Culling open and late-calving cows should be seriously considered because these cows are at higher risk for being infected or acting as carriers of the disease.
- Create high- and low-risk herds. Virgin heifers and cows unlikely to have been exposed to *T foetus* should be classified as low-risk herds [17]. Addition of cattle to the low-risk groups should only be done if you can verify the disease-free status of these animals.
- Any cow that aborts or has a uterine discharge should be isolated and cultured for the presence of disease. If not culled, they should be placed in the high-risk herd and given sexual rest.
- Vaccination of all herd females with an approved trichomonosis vaccine is an important tool in reducing the pregnancy wastage that accompanies the disease. Currently *TrichGuard* (Fort Dodge) is the only commercially available United States Department of Agriculture–licensed

product for use in the control of this disease in the United States. This proprietary vaccine is a Freund adjuvant killed protozoal-derived vaccine. It requires two subcutaneous injections 2 to 4 weeks apart with the last injection given 4 weeks before the beginning of the breeding season. Each subsequent year all cows should receive a single booster injection 4 weeks before the beginning of the breeding season to promote an immune response. All new cattle and heifers must receive the two injection series before the breeding season. The vaccine does not prevent infection or disease but reduces the severity and duration of disease. There seems to be no benefit to the vaccination of bulls [74].

- Artificial insemination, using semen from reputable bull studs, reduces the chance of infected breeding contacts. This practice may be a less practical tool in many commercial beef cattle operations, but is known to be an effective control tool [17].

Control strategies vary from herd to herd. Many factors must be considered when planning a control program. Periodic assessment of a *T foetus* control program is advisable.

Summary

T foetus is a venereal disease of cattle that has a clear pattern of adverse reproductive sequela in affected females with a carrier state in the bull in which he shows no outward signs. Given sexual rest and symptomatic treatment, the female returns to reproductive viability. In contrast, the male remains infective and is a risk to other female contacts. Prevention of the disease relies on excluding infected males and females from the population of susceptible cattle. Control of this disease requires a diagnostic plan to identify, isolate, and treat infected females and eliminate or cull infected males. Advances in diagnostics, using improvements in culture technique and the application of newer methods, such as PCR, enhance the likelihood of detecting infected animals.

References

[1] Morgan BB. Bovine trichomoniasis. Minneapolis: Burgess Publishing Co.; 1946.

[2] Emmerson M. Trichomoniasis in cattle. J Am Vet Med Assoc 1932;34:636–40.

[3] BonDurant RH, Honigberg BM. Trichomonads of veterinary importance. In: Kreier JP, editor. Parasitic protozoa, volume 9. 2nd edition. San Diego, CA: Academic Press, Inc.; 1994. p. 136–62.

[4] Levine ND. Protozoan parasites of domestic animals and of man. 1st edition. Minneapolis: Burgess; 1985. p. 59–79.

[5] Adl SM, Simpson AGB, Farmer MA, et al. The new higher level classification of Eukaryotes with emphasis on the taxonomy of Protists. J Eukaryot Microbiol 2005;52:399–451.

[6] Dennet DP, Reece RL, Barasa JO, et al. Observations on the incidence and distribution of serotypes of *Trictrichomonas foetus* in beef cattle in North-Eastern Australia. Aust Vet J 1974;50:427–31.

[7] Hall MR, Huang J-C, Ota R, et al. Characterization of *Tritrichomonas foetus* antigens, using bovine antiserum. Am J Vet Res 1986;47:2549–53.
[8] Huang JC, Hanks D, Kvasnicka W, et al. Antigentic relationships among field plates of *Tritrichomonas foetus* from cattle. Am J Vet Res 1989;50:1064–8.
[9] Switzer WP. Atrophic rhinitis and trichomonads. Veterinary Medicine 1951;46:478–81.
[10] Fitzgerald PR, Johnson AE, Thorne JL, et al. Experimental infections of the bovine genital system with trichomonads from the digestive tracts of swine. Am J Vet Res 1958;19:775–9.
[11] Jensen EA, Hammond DM. A morphological study of trichomonads and related flagellates from the bovine digestive tract. J Protozool 1964;11:386–94.
[12] Felleisen RSJ, Lambelet N, Bachmann P, et al. Detection of *Tritrichomonas foetus* by PCR and DNA enzyme immunoassay based on rRNA gene unit sequences. J Clin Microbiol 1998; 36:513–9.
[13] Hammond DM, Bartlett DE. The distribution of *Trichomonas foetus* in the preputial cavity of infected bulls. Am J Vet Res 1943;4:143–9.
[14] Parsonson IM, Clark BL, Dufty JH. The pathogenesis of *Tritrichomonas foetus* infection in the bull. Aust Vet J 1974;50:421–3.
[15] Roberts SJ. Infections diseases caused by infertility in cows. In: Roberts SJ, editor. Veterinary obstetrics and genital diseases. 3rd edition. Ann Arbor, MI: Edward Bros, Inc.; 1986. p. 147.
[16] Anderson ML, Barr BC, Conrad PA. Protozoal causes of reproductive failure in domestic ruminants. Vet Clin North Am Food Anim Pract 1994;10:439–61.
[17] Peter D. Bovine venereal diseases. In: Younguist RB, editor. Current therapy in large animal theriogenology. Philadelphia: WB Saunders Co.; 1997. p. 355–63.
[18] Clark BL, Parsonson IM, Dufty JH. Experimental infection of bulls with *Tritrichomonas foetus*. Aust Vet J 1974;50(5):189–91.
[19] Christensen HR, Clark BL, Parsonson IM. Incidence of *Tritrichomonas foetus* in young replacement bulls following introduction into an infected herd. Aust Vet J 1977;53:132–4.
[20] Christensen HR, Clark BL. Spread of *Tritrichomonas foetus* in beef bulls in an infected herd. Aust Vet J 1979;55(4):205.
[21] Skirrow SZ, BonDurant RH, Farley J, et al. Efficacy of ipronidazole against trichomoniasis in beef bulls. J Am Vet Med Assoc 1985;187:405–7.
[22] BonDurant RH, Anderson ML, Blanchard P, et al. Prevalence of trichomoniasis among California beef herds. J Am Vet Assoc 1990;196:1590–3.
[23] Rae DO, Chenoweth PJ, Genho PC, et al. Prevalence of *Tritrichomonas fetus* in a bull population and effect on production in a large cow-calf enterprise. J Am Vet Med Assoc 1999; 214:1051–5.
[24] Rae DO, Crews JE, Griener EC, et al. Epidemiology of *Tritrichomonas foetus* in beef bull populations in Florida. Therio 2004;61:605–18.
[25] Abbitt B, Meyerholz GW. *Trichomonas foetus* infection of range bulls in South Florida. Vet Med Sm Anim Clin 1979;74:1339–42.
[26] Clark BL, Dufty JH, Parsonson RDA, et al. Studies on the transmission of *Tritrichomonas foetus*. Aust Vet J 1977;53:170–2.
[27] BonDurant RH. Diagnosis, treatment, and control of bovine trichomoniasis. The Compendium on Continuing Education. 1985;7: S179–88.
[28] Clark BL, Dufty JH, Parsonson IM. The effect of *Tritrichomonas foetus* on calving rates in beef cattle. Austr Vet J 1983;60(3):71–4.
[29] Parsonson IM, Clark BL, Dufty JH. Early pathogenesis and pathology of *Tritrichomonas foetus* infection in virgin heifers. J Comp Pathol 1976;86:59–66.
[30] Alexander GI. An outbreak of bovine trichomoniasis in Queensland and its control. Aust Vet J 1953;29:61–9.
[31] Skirrow SZ, BonDurant RH. Induced *Tritrichomonas foetus* infection in beef heifers. J Am Vet Med Assoc 1990;196:885–9.
[32] Kimsey PB. Bovine trichomoniasis. In: Morrow DA, editor. Current therapy in theriogenology. 2nd edition. Philadelphia: WB Saunders Co; 1986; p. 275–9.

[33] Skirrow SZ. Identification of trichomonad carrier cows. J Am Vet Med Assoc 1987;191: 553–4.
[34] Rhyan JC, Stackhouse LL, Quinn WJ. Fetal and placental lesions in bovine abortion due to *Tritrichomonas foetus*. Vet Pathol 1988;25:350–5.
[35] Rhyan JC, Blanchard PC, Kvasnicka WG, et al. Tissue-invasive *Tritrichomonas foetus* in four aborted fetuses. J Vet Diagn Invest 1995;7:409–12.
[36] Burgess DE, Knoblock KF, Daughtery T, et al. Cytotoxic and hemolytic effect of *Tritrichomonas foetus* on mammalian cells. Infect Immun 1990;58:3627–32.
[37] Burgess DE, McDonald D. Analysis of adhesions and cytotoxicity of *Tritrichomonas foetus* to mammalian cells by use of monoclonal antibodies. Infect Immun 1992;60:4253–9.
[38] Kreiger JN, Ravdin JI, Rein MF. Contact-dependent cytopathogenic mechanism of *Trichomonas vaginalis*. Infect Immun 1985;50:778–86.
[39] Aydintug MK, Leid RW, Widders PR. Antibody enhances killing of *Tritrichomonas foetus* by the alternative bovine complement pathway. Infect Immun 1990;58:944–8.
[40] Aydintug MK, Widders PR, Leid RW. Bovine polymorphonuclear leukocyte killing of *Tritrichomonas foetus*. Infect Immun 1993;61:2995–3002.
[41] Rae DO. Impact of trichomoniasis on the cow-calf producer's profitability. J Am Vet Med Assoc 1989;194:771–5.
[42] Speer CA, White MW. Bovine trichomoniasis. Better diagnostics and control could save beef industry $650 million annually. Large Anim Vet 1991;46:18–20.
[43] Wilson SK, Kocan AA, Gaudy ET, et al. The prevalence of trichomoniasis in Okalahoma beef bulls. Bovine Pract 1979;14:109–10.
[44] Fitzgerald PR, Johnson AE, Thorne JL, et al. Trichomoniasis in range cattle. Veterinary Medicine 1958;53:249–52.
[45] Wikse SE. Investigation of impaired fertility in beef cattle herds. In: The North American veterinary conference proceedings. Gainesville (FL): Eastern States Veterinary Association; 1995. p. 503–4.
[46] Bondurant RH, van Hoosear KA, Corbeil LB, et al. Serological response to in vitro-shed antigen(s) of Tritrichomonas foetus in cattle. Clin Diagn Lab Immunol 1996;3:432–7.
[47] Taylor MA, Marshall RN, Stack M. Morphological differentiation of *Tritrichomonas foetus* from other protozoa of the bovine reproductive tract. Br Vet J 1994;150:73–80.
[48] BonDurant RH, Gajadhar A, Campero CM, et al. Preliminary characterization of a *Tritrichomonas foetus*-like protozoan isolated from preputial smegma of virgin bulls. Bov Pract 1999;33:124–7.
[49] Groteluschen DM, Cheney J, Hudson DB, et al. Bovine trichomoniasis: results of a slaughter survey in Colorado and Nebraska. Theriogenology 1994;42:165–71.
[50] Johnson AE. The diagnosis of trichomoniasis in the bull. Proc of the US Livestock Sanitary Assoc 1965;69:183–9.
[51] Tedesco LF, Errico F, Baglivi LP. Diagnosis of Tritrichomonas foetus infection in bulls using two sampling mehtods and a trasnsport medium. Austr Vet J 1979;55:322–4.
[52] Skirrow SZ, BonDurant RH. Bovine trichomoniasis. Vet Bull 1988;58:592–603.
[53] BonDurant RH. Abortion/infertility caused by *Tritrichomonas foetus*. In: Kirkbride CA, editor. Laboratory diagnosis of livestock abortion. Ames, IA: Iowa State University Press; 1990. p. 161–4.
[54] Appell LH, Mickelsen WD, Thomas MW, et al. A comparison of techniques used for the diagnosis of *Tritrichomonas foetus* infections in beef bulls. Agri-Practice 1993;14:30–4.
[55] Schönmann MJ, BonDurant RH, Gardner IA, et al. Comparison sampling and culture methods for the diagnosis of *Tritrichomonas foetus* infection in bulls. Vet Record 1994; 134:620–3.
[56] Diamond LS. Lumen-dwelling protozoa: entamoeba, trichomnads, and giardia. In: Jensen JB, editor. In vitro cultivation of protozoan parasites. Boca Raton, FL: CRC Press; 1983. p. 65–109.

[57] Bryan LA, Campbell JR, Gajadhar AA. Effects of temperature on the survival of *Tritrichomonas foetus* in transport, Diamond's and InPouch TF media. Vet Rec 1999;144:227–32.
[58] Borchardt KA, Norman BB, Thomas MW, et al. Evaluation of a new culture method for diagnosing *Tritrichomonas foetus* infection. Vet Med 1992;87:104–12.
[59] Fitzgerald PR, Hammond DM, Miner MC, et al. Relative efficacy of various methods of obtaining preputial samples for diagnosis of trichomoniasis in bulls. Am J Vet Res 1952; 13:452–7.
[60] Mickelsen WD. Diagnosis of trichomoniasis: herd history and culture techniques. Proc Am Assoc Bovine Pract 1982;15:134–5.
[61] Goodger WJ, Skirrow SZ. Epidemiologic and economic analysis of an unusually long epizootic of trichomoniasis in a large California dairy herd. J Am Vet Med Assoc 1986;189:772–6.
[62] Kittel DR, Campero C, Van Hoosen KA, et al. Comparison of diagnostic methods for detection of active infection with *Tritrichomonas foetus* in beef heifers. J Am Vet Med Assoc 1998;213:519–22.
[63] Speer CA, Severson WE, Cranston HJ, et al. A diagnostic DNA assay for trichomoniasis in cattle. In: Proceedings of the Livestock Conservation Institute, Madison, WI. 1992. p. 128–37.
[64] Ho MSY, Conrad PA, Conrad PJ, et al. Detection of bovine trichomoniasis with a specific DNA probe and polymerase chain reaction amplification system. J Clin Micorobiol 1994;32: 98–104.
[65] Felleisen RSJ. Comparative genetic analysis of tritrchomonadid protozoa by the random amplified polymorphic DNA technique. Parasitol Res 1998;84:153–6.
[66] Mukhufhi N, Irons PC, Michel A, et al. Evaluation of a PCR test for the diagnosis of *Tritrichomonas foetus* infection in bulls: effects of sample collection method, storage and transport medium on the test. Theriogenology 2003;60:1269–78.
[67] Nickel DD, Olson ME, Schultz GA. An improved polymerase chain reaction assay for the detection of *Tritrichomonas foetus* in cattle. Can Vet J 2002;43:213–6.
[68] Campero CM, Dubra CR, Bolondi A, et al. Two-step (culture and PCR) diagnostic approach for differentiation of non-*T. foetus* trichomonads from genitalia of virgin beef bulls in Argentina. Vet Parasitol 2003;112:167–75.
[69] Parker S, Campbell J, McIntosh K, Gajadhar A. Diagnosis of trichomoniasis in 'virgin' bulls by culture and polymerase chain reaction. Can Vet J 2003;44:732–4.
[70] Grahn RA, BonDurant RH, van Hoosear KA, et al. An improved molecular assay for *Tritrichomonas foetus*. Vet Parasitol 2005;127:33–41.
[71] Mutto AA, Giambiaggi S, Angel SO. PCR detection of *Tritrichomonas foetus* in preputial bull fluid without prior DNA isolation. Vet Parasitol 2006;136:357–61. Epub 2005 Dec 28.
[72] Richey EJ. Simple strategies; facilitating veterinarian and producer communication. Large Anim Vet 1991;Mar-Apr:15–8.
[73] Gay JM, Ebel ED, Kearley WP. Comingled grazing as a risk factor for trichomoniasis in beef herds. J Am Vet Med Assoc 1996;209:643–6.
[74] Kvasnicka WG, Hall MR, Hanks DR. Bovine trichomoniasis. In: Howard JL, editor. Current veterinary therapy 4: food animal practice. Philadelphia: WB Saunders Co.; 1999. p. 420–5.
[75] Kimsey PB, Darian BJ, Kendrick JW, et al. Bovine trichomoniasis: diagnosis and treatment. J Am Vet Med Assoc 1980;177:615–9.
[76] McLaughlin DK. Dimetridazole, a systemic treatment for bovine venereal trichomoniasis, III. Trials with cows. J Parasitol 1970;56:39–40.

ELSEVIER
SAUNDERS

Vet Clin Food Anim
22 (2006) 613–621

VETERINARY
CLINICS
Food Animal Practice

Ruminant Coccidiosis

William R. Jolley, MSc, PhD[a,b,*],
Katherine D. Bardsley, MSc[b]

[a]*Department of Veterinary Sciences, University of Wyoming, WY, USA*
[b]*Diagnostic Parasitology and Clinical Pathology Sections, Wyoming State Veterinary Laboratory, 1174 Snowy Range Road, Laramie, WY 82070, USA*

Nearly all vertebrate animals host one or more species of the protozoan parasites that produce the infection referred to as coccidiiasis or coccidiosis. Thousands of coccidian species of herbivorous, omnivorous, and carnivorous animals have been described, and many more exist that remain unnamed. Some cause serious disease, whereas others are of minor or no clinical importance. Producers, veterinarians, and biologists involved in production, health care, and management of ruminant animals usually recognize bloody diarrhea as a common indication of coccidiosis (Fig. 1). Although some of the most pathogenic coccidial infections are a common cause of "bloody scours," nonbloody diarrhea, or "white scours," may also indicate coccidiosis.

The agents that cause coccidiosis are single-celled protozoan organisms that develop inside intestinal cells of their animal hosts. Because their intracellular development results in destruction of the cells in which they multiply, they are all considered parasitic, whether or not they cause disease. Most species that infect ruminants cause no symptoms, even though they may be found in large numbers by standard diagnostic analysis; consequently, distinction between pathogenic species and those of minor clinical importance is essential to differentiating coccidial from viral, bacterial, or other causes of enteric disease.

All of the agents discussed in this article are taxonomically grouped as follows: genus *Eimeria*, family Eimeriidae, order Eucoccidiorida, class Sporozoasida, phylum Apicomplexa. From these taxa come the terms commonly used to identify the organisms or the clinical conditions they cause: eimeriiasis/coccidiiasis (nonpathogenic infection with species in the genus/order),

* Corresponding author. Department of Veterinary Sciences, Wyoming State Veterinary Laboratory, 1174 Snowy Range Road, Laramie, WY 82070.

E-mail address: willjo@uwyo.edu (W.R. Jolley).

doi:10.1016/j.cvfa.2006.07.004

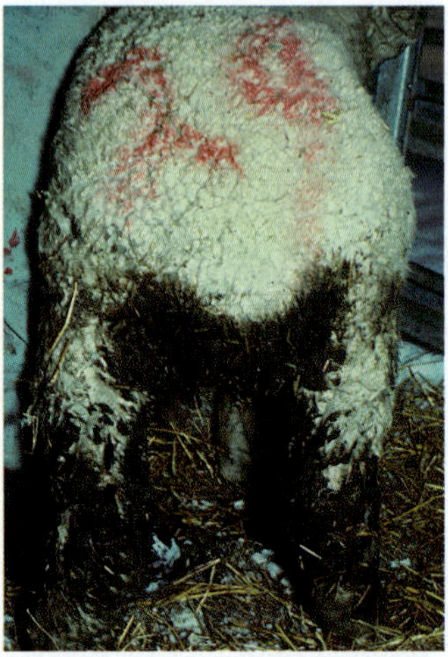

Fig. 1. Patent coccidiosis in a yearling lamb. Referred to by producers as "bloody scours" or "bloody crotch"; the primary causative species in this case was *Eimeria ovinoidalis*. (*Courtesy of* R.C. Bergstrom, Laramie, Wyoming.)

eimeriosis/coccidiosis (pathogenic infection with species in the genus/order), and sporozoa/sporozoan (a spore-forming protozoan animal). Nearly all of the *Eimeria* species of ruminants are rigidly host specific, able to complete development and reproduction in the digestive tract of specific, genetically compatible host species. Detailed information regarding history, taxonomy, host and site specificity, species identification, life cycles and development, ultrastructure, cytochemistry and biochemistry, physiology, cultivation, pathology and pathogenicity, immunology, genetics, control, chemotherapy, and drug resistance is available in several excellent textbooks [1–4].

Estimates of worldwide yearly economic consequences of coccidiosis in cattle and bison were 731 million United States dollars in 1980 [5]; more recently, $400 million was the proposed figure [6]. Factors considered in the loss estimates included mortality, growth retardation, permanent stunting, veterinary expenses, and treatment of clinical coccidiosis. Losses due to subtle impaired development and growth, retarded feed conversion, and other effects of mild or subclinical coccidiosis have not been accurately estimated.

Life cycle

The *Eimeria* species of ruminants develop in a three-stage direct life cycle. Two stages develop within intestinal cells of a host and are referred to as schizogony or merogony and gamogony or gametogony. The third stage, sporogony/sporulation, occurs outside the body of the host in an oocyst that protects encysted, infective sporozoites from lethal environmental conditions. For brevity, the stages will be referred to hereafter as merogony, gamogony, and sporogony.

Merogony involves two or more cycles in which merozoites are produced by multiple asexual fission. After maturation of the meronts, the parasitized host cell ruptures, releasing merozoites that enter other cells and repeat the cycle or progress to gamogony. Gamogony constitutes the sexual stage of development, which is the terminal stage in a host. Gamogony begins when merozoites produced in the final phase of merogony enter cells and produce either macrogamonts or microgamonts, which mature to macrogametes and microgametes, respectively. Macrogametes are somewhat analogous to mammalian ova, and microgametes to sperm. Flagellated microgametes liberated from host cells enter cells containing a macrogamete and fertilize the macrogamete to produce a zygote. An impermeable cyst wall forms around the zygote, after which it is known as an oocyst, which is then discharged from the host cell into the lumen of the intestine and passes from the host in feces.

Sporogony is the "ripening" or development to infectivity of the oocyst, when exposed to mild temperatures, oxygen, and moist environmental conditions. The sporulated, infective oocyst of *Eimeria* species contains four subcysts called sporocysts, each of which contains two sporozoites, for a total of eight basic infective units in each oocyst. Infection of a host begins when feces containing infectious oocysts are ingested with contaminated food or water. Digestive enzymes in the newly infected host break down the impermeability of the oocysts and sporocysts and activate the sporozoites, enabling them to excyst and initiate the asexual phase of development [1–4].

Completion of the cycle from the beginning of merogony to the release of newly produced oocysts requires approximately 14 to 21 days, depending on the species of *Eimeria* and the host. Clinical coccidiosis usually occurs during the late stages of gamogony, when oocysts are forming and being discharged into the intestinal lumen.

Oocyst passage from onset to completion is referred to as the patent period of infection and spans approximately 3 to 10 days, depending on coccidian species, host species, infectious dose of oocysts, condition and age of host, and other factors. Initial cycles of merogony normally begin in the lower duodenum or jejunum of a host and progress further down the intestine with each successive cycle. Gamogony may occur in the lower ileum or in the cecum and colon.

Epidemiology

Infective oocysts are present in the soil, vegetation, or water sources of virtually all sites inhabited by ruminants. After sporogony, the oocysts are capable of surviving and retaining infectivity for weeks or months, depending on environmental conditions. Dry conditions compounded by heat or extreme cold shorten the infective life-span of oocysts, although they have been shown to survive lengthy winter seasons under an insulating blanket of snow or in layers of dung, soil, or vegetation. Moderate temperatures, air exposure, and moist environmental conditions facilitate sporogony and enhance the survival and viability of oocysts.

Regular infections with a mixture of pathogenic and nonpathogenic coccidian species occur throughout the lives of mature animals and provide oocyst contamination transmissible to young animals. Mixed infections with three to five species of pathogenic or nonpathogenic coccidia are normal. Most ruminants older than 1 year have acquired significant species-specific protective immunity from initial infections with pathogenic species. The immunity is not absolute, but it will prevent clinical episodes of the magnitude of the initial infection. Individual pathogenic species of *Eimeria* may sicken a host alone or in concert with one or more others but seldom cause disease twice in a healthy, normal host.

Coccidiosis usually appears in areas crowded with animals, such as feedlots, small pastures, and shady creek bottoms during hot summer weather, or near water tanks, hay stacks, or salt licks. Adult animals passing a "normal" number of oocysts in crowded conditions steadily raise oocyst contamination to a level hazardous to susceptible calves, fawns, lambs, or kids. Young, patently infected, confined animals quickly increase oocyst contamination to extreme levels, after which other young, immunologically naïve animals are at high risk for serious disease when placed in those heavily contaminated facilities. Stressful events such as weaning, crowding, shipping, food changes, nutritional deficiencies, concomitant infections with other parasitic agents, and weather events, such as blizzards or excessively hot temperatures, appear to facilitate the development of clinical coccidiosis. Correlation between stress and clinical coccidiosis is considered somewhat subjective but is widely believed to enhance outbreak predictability. Coccidiosis is an annual event in many ranching and other livestock production operations, sometimes reliably timed to a particular period [7–10].

Pathobiology

Few species of the coccidian parasites of ruminants cause significant disease; for example, only *Eimeria bovis* and *E zuernii* of 13 or more species in cattle and bison are primary causes of life-threatening coccidiosis, with *E auburnensis* and *E alabamensis* being only moderately pathogenic [4,7]. Of 16 species in domestic Rocky Mountain bighorn, mouflon, or other sheep, *E ahsata, E ovinoidalis,* and *E bakuensis* (*ovina*) are considered serious pathogens [4,10]. In goats, 15 species have been described, of which *E christenseni*, *E arloingi*, *E caprina*, and *E ninakohlyakimovae* are of major concern [4,8].

Mechanisms and degree of damage depend on the species of *Eimeria* involved, the size of the infective dose of oocysts, stress, and various host-related factors, including age, physical condition, genetic susceptibility, and the degree of immunity that has developed from previous low levels of infection [2–4,7]. Clinical signs of coccidiosis are nearly always caused by gamont and oocyst development in the lower ileum, cecum, and colon. Most intestinal coccidia develop in epithelial cells of the lamina propria; a few exceptions include the first meront of *E bovis* in endothelial cells in the lacteals of the villi in the lower ileum of calves and the meronts found in histologic sections of intestinal lymph nodes of some sheep.

Damage from the gamogony-related cycle at the onset of patency includes mucosal destruction and erosion, usually in the lower ilium, cecum, and colon [11–17]. Petechial hemorrhage is common in mild clinical cases, with diffuse hemorrhage occurring in more extreme coccidiosis. A bloody semiliquid accumulates in the lower digestive tract early in the patent period, when numerous oocysts, fibrin, and tissue fragments are released from the mucosa. White patches or lines and other gray, brown, or pink-shaded areas may be visible on the mucosal surface at necropsy [4,14]. In some areas the submucosa may also be destroyed, after which a membrane eventually forms over the damaged area. Depending on the severity of damage and whether the infected animal survives, partial or complete tissue repair and recovery may occur.

A condition referred to as nervous coccidiosis sometimes affects cattle, soon to long after clinical coccidiosis caused by *E zuernii* [7,18]. It is more often seen in animals 6 months or more of age than in younger calves. Affected animals spontaneously fall to the ground and begin a spasmodic, bicyclic type of leg movement, with contraction of the dorsal muscles of the neck and back, causing the head to be drawn dorsoposteriorly. After a period of several minutes, they spontaneously recover, rise, and resume apparently normal function. The physiologic cause of the condition is unknown, but it is believed to be related to plasma electrolyte imbalance. Animals with this condition may display the symptoms for months after apparent recovery from patent coccidiosis [19].

Diagnosis

Young animals beginning to show diarrhea, dysentery, anemia, dehydration, weakness, anorexia, and emaciation, with or without respiratory distress, should be suspected of having and be examined for coccidiosis. Microscopic examination of diarrheic or bloody feces from young animals remains the most direct, definitive, and cost-effective method of diagnosis [4,7]. Serologic analytical methods by ELISA and Western Blot have been developed, but they are not as definitive as visual examination of feces [7]. Traditional fecal analysis involves concentration of oocysts from feces by a sugar or salt flotation method, followed by identification of species by microscopic differentiation of the concentrated oocysts (Fig. 2) [1–4,7].

Diarrheic discharge, usually bloodless, from viral, bacterial, or other causes, sometimes contains moderate to large numbers of oocysts of

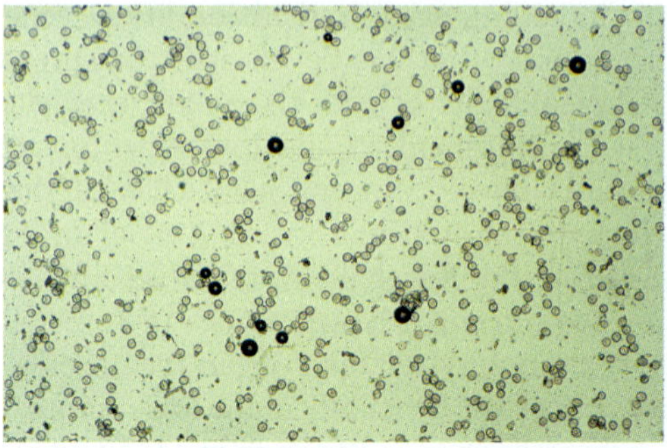

Fig. 2. Diagnostic fecal flotation from a calf with patent coccidiosis due to *Eimeria zuernii*. Oocyst count is 325,000 oocysts per gram of feces. Dark spots are air bubbles. (Original magnification ×100.) (*Courtesy of* W.R. Jolley, MSc, PhD, Laramie, Wyoming.)

nonpathogenic *Eimeria* species. In these situations, identification of the coccidia in fecal specimens is essential to accurate diagnosis of the clinical problem, which may be unrelated to the protozoa.

Oocysts are most numerous in feces or tissues discharged in early patency and remain at high numbers for approximately 3 to 7 days, after which the entire endogenous cycle is completed, and fecal oocyst counts often drop to zero. Because of the disappearance of oocysts from feces soon after the onset of patency, timely collection of fecal samples for diagnostic testing is important. Feces for diagnostic analysis should be collected from animals at the beginning of a diarrheic phase, rather than a week or two after onset. If the host survives the clinical infection and begins to recover, "normal" subclinical infections may not begin again for weeks or months. Occasionally, oocysts will not be found in fluid, blood, or fecal discharge from animals with patent infections. In those cases, excreted tissue and fibrin fragments, or tissue scrapings from the intestinal mucosa of a dead animal, should be examined in a wet mount by light microscopy. Any or all stages of gamogony will be visible in cells of those tissue fragments if the infection is coccidial [14]. During the normal course of infection through a herd, patency will progress from a few animals infected initially through other herd mates over time, after which survivors will recover partially or completely. Feces taken for diagnosis should be collected from several animals at the beginning of a diarrheic phase, because members of the herd that have scoured for 3 or more days may pass few or no oocysts.

Eimerian coccidiosis is seldom seen in animals less than 3 weeks of age, because the prepatent periods range from approximately 15 to 21 days. Although some infections begin during the first week of life, most occur later, unless oocyst contamination in the birthing area is excessive. A somewhat distant relative of the eimerian coccidia, *Cryptosporidium parvum* (discussed elsewhere in this issue), is capable of producing diarrhea within a week of birth in newborn animals of many different species. Cryptosporidiosis and eimerian coccidiosis are sometimes considered one disease, even though their diagnosis, pathogenesis, host specificity, and control methods differ significantly.

Control

Prevention is the key to controlling coccidiosis. Effective strategies include minimizing exposure of susceptible young animals to infective oocysts and administration of prophylactic coccidiostatic drugs to infected animals during asexual developmental stages [4,18–29]. After intracellular formation of oocysts has begun, they are impermeable to drugs and most other chemicals. Supportive care may minimize death loss by preventing dehydration, secondary infections, nutritional deprivation, and exposure to temperature extremes.

Sanitation efforts intended to eliminate or reduce oocyst intake related to the build-up of fecal contamination have had limited success. Animals on range often avoid clinical-level exposure until round-up and movement to relatively small pastures, pens, or feedlots, although periods of extreme heat or cold may cause animals to collect in areas near streams, buildings, or treed shelters. Small facilities with slatted floors, water tanks with overflow prevention control, and elevated feed bunks designed to minimize oocyst intake from ground-level feeding or drinking are somewhat effective.

Numerous anticoccidial drugs have been developed, tested, and used to prevent or reduce ruminant production losses, but none is 100% effective. Some of those used for control of avian coccidiosis are too toxic for use in ruminants. Amprolium, decoquinate, lasalocid, lincomycin, monensin, and salinomycin are commonly used in calves, fawns, lambs, and kids. They affect the early stages of development, including sporozoites, meronts, and merozoites, and are normally applied with water (amprolium) or feed during a period when coccidiosis is predictable, based on historical occurrences. These coccidiostatic prophylactics do not completely prevent development of the agents, but they normally reduce infection to a subclinical level. When the drugs are administered at an effective level during the period of infection, a protective level of immunity to the species involved develops, after which the medication may be discontinued with significant protection against reinfection by the initial agents.

Treatment of animals during unpredictable or spontaneous patency with a sulfonamide or a benzene acetonitrile compound (BAC) may be warranted. The sulfonamides have limited efficacy against the coccidia but are effective against secondary bacterial agents that cause pneumonia, which is especially significant in calves with *E zuernii* or *E bovis* infections. Two of the BACs, diclazuril and toltazuril, when administered orally as a single dose within a week of patency, effectively controlled coccidiosis in calves. When these are applied to animals early in a spontaneous or unexpected outbreak, clinical coccidiosis may be suppressed in infected herd members approaching patency.

Some species of coccidia have developed resistance to coccidiostats used repeatedly for long periods, especially in poultry production. Use of coccidiostatic drugs in ruminant animal production tends to be periodic, rather than continuous as in poultry production, and reports of drug resistance are limited.

Development and testing of vaccines have been and are ongoing. The process has frequently involved inefficient, expensive procedures, including production and collection of oocysts from host animals, attempts to alter the infectivity or pathogenicity of oocyst-encased sporozoites, determination and administration of immunity-stimulating but nonpathogenic doses of oocysts, and other logistical issues. Vaccine use for control of bovine coccidiosis is not currently significant.

Wise management decisions based on knowledge of basic biology, epidemiology, diagnosis, and control of ruminant coccidiosis will increase production, production efficiency, and profit. Information about the disease and currently effective methods of preventing significant loss is widely available.

References

[1] Pellerdy LP. Coccidia and coccidiosis. Budapest (Hungary): Akademiai Kiado; 1965.

[2] Hammond DM, Long PL. The coccidia: Eimeria, Isospora, Toxoplasma and related genera. Baltimore (MD): University Park Press; 1973.

[3] Long PL. The biology of the coccidia. Baltimore (MD): University Park Press; 1982.

[4] Levine ND. Veterinary protozoology. Ames (IA): Iowa State University Press; 1985.

[5] Fitzgerald PR. The economic impact of coccidiosis in domestic animals. Adv Vet Sci Comp Med 1980;24:121–43.

[6] Matjila PT, Penzhorn BL. Occurrence and diversity of bovine coccidian at three localities in South Africa. Vet Parasitol 2002;104:93–102.

[7] Dougschies A, Najdrowski M. Eimeriosis in cattle: current understanding. Journal of Veterinary Medicine 2005;52:417–27.

[8] Norton CC. Coccidia of the domestic goat *Capra hircus*, with notes on *Eimeria ovinoidalis* and *E. bakuensis* (syn. *E. ovina*) from the sheep *Ovis aries*. Parasitol 1986;92:279–89.

[9] Faber JE, Kollmann D, Heise A, et al. *Eimeria* infections in cows in the periparturient phase and their calves: oocyst excretion and levels of specific serum and colostrum antibodies. Vet Parasitol 2002;104:1–17.

[10] Reeg KJ, Gauly M, Bauer C, et al. Coccidial infections in housed lambs: oocyst excretion, antibody levels and genetic influences on the infection. Vet Parasitol 2005;127:209–19.

[11] Friend SCE, Stockdale PHG. Experimental Eimeria bovis infections in calves: a histopathologic study. Can J Comp Med 1980;44:129–40.

[12] Gregory MW, Catchpole J. Ovine coccidiosis: the pathology of Eimeria crandalis infection. Int J Parasitol 1990;20:849–60.

[13] Heath HL, Blagburn BL, Elsasser TH, et al. Hormonal modulation of the physiologic responses of calves infected with Eimeria bovis. Am J Vet Res 1997;58:891–6.

[14] Gardiner CH, Fayer R, Dubey JP. An atlas of protozoan parasites in animal tissues. 2nd edition. Washington, DC: Armed Forces Institute of Pathology; 1998. p. 1–84.

[15] Aleksandersen M, Lie KI, Gjerde B, et al. Lymphocyte depletion in ileal Peyer's patch follicles in lambs infected with *Eimeria ovinoidalis*. Clin Diagn Lab Immunol 2002;9:83–91.

[16] Mundt HC, Bangoura B, Rinke M, et al. Pathology and treatment of *Eimeria zuernii* in calves: investigations in an infection model. Int J Parasitol 2005;54:223–30.

[17] Dai YB, Liu XY, Liu M, et al. Pathogenic effects of the coccidium Eimeria ninakohlyakimovae in goats. Vet Res Commun 2006;30:149–60.
[18] Sato J, Nitanai A, Kurosawa T, et al. Anticoccidial efficacy of medium-chain triglycerides (MCT) in calves. J Vet Med Sci 2004;66:1583–5.
[19] Jolley WR, Bergstrom RC. Research and diagnostic data 1975–1995 (unpublished).
[20] Benz GW, Ernst JV. Efficacy of salinomycin in treatment of experimental Eimeria bovis infections in calves. Am J Vet Res 1979;40:1180–6.
[21] Stockdale PH, Sheard A, Tiffin GB. Resistance to *Eimeria bovis* produced after chemotherapy of experimental infections in calves. Vet Parasitol 1983;9:171–7.
[22] Fitzgerald PR, Mansfield ME. Control of bovine coccidiosis with monensin in nonresistant newborn calves. Am J Vet Res 1984;45:1984–8.
[23] Fitzgerald PR, Mansfield ME. Effect of decoquinate on the control of coccidiosis in young ruminating calves. Am J Vet Res 1986;47:130–3.
[24] Foreyt WJ, Rice DH, Wescott RB. Evaluation of lasalocid as a coccidiostat in calves: titration, efficacy and comparison with monensin and decoquinate. Am J Vet Res 1986;47: 2031–5.
[25] Waggoner JK, Cecava MJ, Kazacos KR. Efficacy of lasalocid and decoquinate against coccidiosis in naturally infected dairy calves. J Dairy Sci 1994;77:349–53.
[26] McMeniman NP, Elliot R. Control of coccidia in young calves using lasalocid. Aust Vet J 1995;72:7–9.
[27] Quigley JD, Drewry JJ, Murray LM, et al. Effects of lasalocid in milk replacer or calf starter on health and performance of calves challenged with Eimeria species. J Dairy Sci 1997;80: 2972–6.
[28] Cox FEG. Control of coccidiosis: lessons from other sporozoa. Int J Parasitol 1998;28: 165–79.
[29] Mundt HC, Daugschies A, Uebe F, et al. Efficacy of toltrazuril against artificial infections with *Eimeria bovis* in calves. Parasitol Res 2003;90:S166–7.

ELSEVIER
SAUNDERS

Vet Clin Food Anim
22 (2006) 623–643

VETERINARY
CLINICS
Food Animal Practice

Giardiasis and Cryptosporidiosis in Ruminants

Ryan M. O'Handley, BSc, PhD[a,b],
Merle E. Olson, DVM, MSc[c,d,e,*]

[a]*Environmental Biotechnology Cooperative Research Centre, School of Veterinary and Biomedical Sciences, Murdoch University, South Street, Murdoch, Western Australia 6164, Australia*
[b]*Department of Health Management, Atlantic Veterinary College, Charlottetown, Prince Edward Island, Canada, C1A 4P3*
[c]*Bow Valley Research, 3707 Underhill Place NW, Calgary, Alberta, Canada, T2N 4G3*
[d]*MBEC Bioproducts, University of Calgary, Calgary, Alberta, Canada, T2N 1N4*
[e]*BioMedical Engineering, University of Alberta, Edmonton, Alberta, Canada, T6G 2V4*

Although differing considerably with respect to their biology, the parasites *Giardia duodenalis* and *Cryptosporidium parvum* have often been discussed collectively because of their role as common causes of waterborne gastrointestinal disease in humans. Because both parasites are extremely common in ruminants, much of the discussion and research concerning *G duodenalis* and *C parvum* during the past decade has focused on their zoonotic potential and the role of ruminants as reservoirs for human infection. By contrast, the importance of these parasites as causes of disease and production losses in ruminants appears to have received little attention. Recent research indicates that, although both *G duodenalis* and *C parvum* infections in ruminants do pose some risk for zoonotic transmission, the risk is much less significant than was once believed and is easily managed. Research also indicates that, although *G duodenalis* is not likely to be a major cause of clinical disease in ruminants, it may have an important and overlooked impact on production. *C parvum*, by contrast, remains an important cause of diarrhea in neonatal ruminants, but it does not appear to be as significant a pathogen in beef calves as it is in dairy calves. In addition, abomasal cryptosporidiosis, caused by *C andersoni*, may be an emerging pathogen of significant economic importance in the beef and dairy cattle industries.

* Corresponding author. Bow Valley Research, 3707 Underhill Place NW, Calgary, Alberta, Canada, T2N 4G3.
E-mail address: molson@ucalgary.ca (M.E. Olson).

doi:10.1016/j.cvfa.2006.07.002

Giardiasis

Giardiasis is a common intestinal disease caused by flagellated protozoan parasites belonging to the genus *Giardia*. Most mammals are susceptible to infection by *G duodenalis*, which is synonymous with *G intestinalis* and *G lamblia*. The parasite is a well-recognized cause of gastrointestinal disease in humans, particularly travelers and children in day-care centers, and it is a frequently identified pathogen in waterborne outbreaks of gastrointestinal disease [1]. In ruminants, *G duodenalis* is one of the most common parasites identified, and a great deal of research has focused on the potential for ruminants, particularly cattle, to act as reservoirs for human outbreaks of giardiasis. However, recent evidence suggests that *G duodenalis* infections in ruminants may not be as important as was once thought with respect to zoonotic transmission and that *G duodenalis* may be an important production-limiting parasite of ruminants.

Life cycle and transmission

Giardia has a simple, direct life cycle: the parasite alternates between a motile feeding trophozoite stage and an infective, environmentally resistant, transmissive stage termed a cyst (Fig. 1). Infection is established when a susceptible host ingests cysts. It is believed that positive hydrogen ions from either gastric acid or bicarbonate secretion trigger excystation and the release of trophozoites. *Giardia* trophozoites multiply asexually by binary fission and rapidly colonize the small intestine. The trophozoites remain extracellular and adhere to the epithelium of the host using a specialized organelle on their ventral surface, termed the adhesive disk (Fig. 2). In ruminants, *Giardia* trophozoites can be found along the entire length of the small intestine, with the greatest number located along the surface of the jejunum [2]. It is likely that cholesterol deprivation induces *Giardia* trophozoites to encyst within the intestine, and the cysts are then voided by the host in the feces.

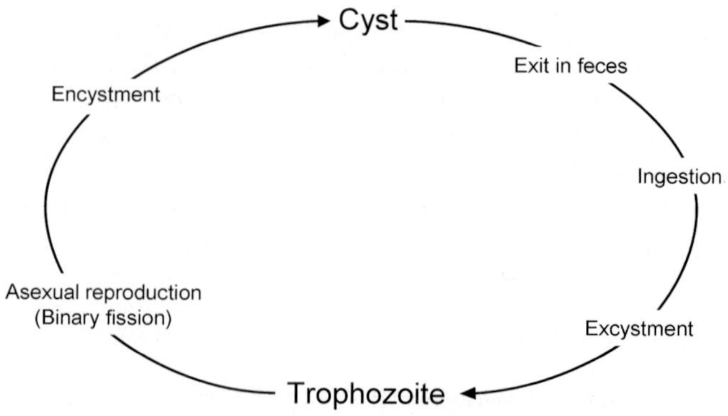

Fig. 1. Life cycle of *Giardia duodenalis*.

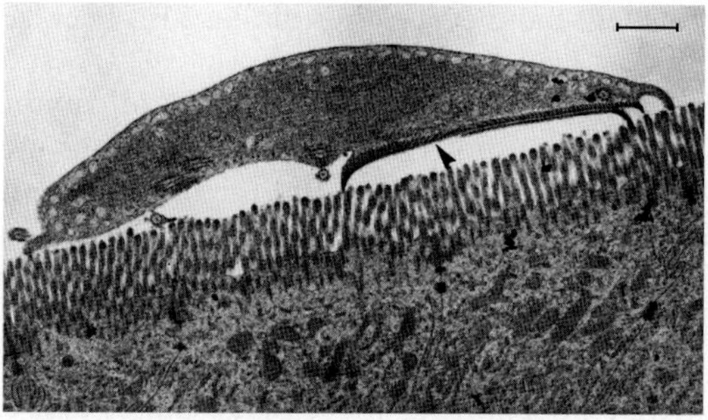

Fig. 2. Transmission electron micrograph (lead stain) of a *G duodenalis* trophozoite in the jejunum of a naturally infected calf. Note the prominent ventral adhesive disk (*arrow*). Bar = 1 μm.

Unlike most other fecally transmitted parasites, which require some time in the environment to become infectious, *Giardia* cysts are immediately infectious after being voided in the feces. Thus transmission occurs readily through direct contact. At the peak of infection, ruminants can excrete 10^6 *G duodenalis* cysts per gram of feces. Cysts remain infectious for months in cool, damp surroundings and rapidly accumulate in environments such as dairies. Because the infectious dose for *G duodenalis* is 10 cysts [3], *Giardia* infection spreads rapidly among ruminants. In addition, cysts are much more resistant than bacteria to disinfection and can survive the levels of chlorination used in water treatment [4]. Hence, outbreaks of giardiasis in the human population are often the result of waterborne transmission [1]. However, ruminants do not appear to play a significant role in transmission of *G duodenalis* to humans (see further discussion).

Epidemiology

The past 15 years have seen a large amount of research examining the epidemiology of giardiasis in ruminants. Results of these studies indicate that *G duodenalis* is one of the most common parasites infecting ruminants worldwide. *G duodenalis* most likely infects all ruminant species and has been reported in cattle [5–8], sheep [9,10], goats [11,12], camels [13], elk, and deer [14]. The prevalence of *G duodenalis* is high in ruminants, and longitudinal studies in both dairy and beef calves indicate that 100% of calves are likely to be infected with *G duodenalis* in the first few months of life [5,6,15]. In sheep, cumulative infection rates of 82% and 94% have been reported in lambs and ewes, respectively, in the United States [16]. However, it is likely that these infection rates were underestimated, because some animals were only examined once. Among pastured lambs in the United Kingdom, nearly 70% excreted *Giardia* cysts at some point during a 9-week study [9]. In goats, a recent study demonstrated a cumulative prevalence of 100% among adult goats during the periparturient period [12]; a rise in periparturient prevalence and cyst excretion has also been reported in sheep and cattle [15,16].

Interestingly, despite the virtual guarantee that all ruminants will be exposed to *G duodenalis* cysts shortly after birth, infections are most common toward the end of the neonatal period, and the infections are chronic. *Giardia* cysts have been detected in ruminants as young as 4 days of age [16]. However, the prepatent period for *G duodenalis* in ruminants ranges from 7 to 8 days for calves [17] to 6 to 10 days for goats [18] and 10 to 21 days for sheep [17]. Therefore, it is likely that cysts observed in 4-day-old calves do not indicate active infection. In most cases, initial cyst excretion occurs a few weeks after birth; the average age observed at initial cyst excretion is approximately 30 days for calves [5,15] and 23 days for lambs [9].

It is not completely understood why *Giardia* infections tend to occur toward the end of the neonatal period, whereas *C parvum* infections, for example, occur earlier in ruminants. It has been proposed that passive immunity initially protects young ruminants from *G duodenalis* infections [19], but definitive studies have yet to be conducted. The actual duration of cyst excretion is not known, but it has been demonstrated that dairy calves can excrete *Giardia* cysts for at least 100 days with no significant decline in prevalence or cyst excretion intensity during that time [5]. In beef calves, cyst excretion for as long as 25 weeks has been reported [15]. Naturally and experimentally infected lambs, along with experimentally infected goats, have been shown to excrete *Giardia* cysts for more than 10 weeks [10,20]. Some studies have indicated a decline in prevalence and cyst excretion intensity in cattle with age [15], suggesting that there is an eventual clearance of the infection. However, recent studies examining older cattle contradict these findings, reporting prevalences of 52% in 1- to 2-year-old heifers [21] and 72% in a herd of adult dairy cows [22]. It is likely that the previously observed reduction in prevalence and cyst excretion may be the result of a dilution effect on cyst excretion by an increase in fecal production in older animals, given that these recent studies examined larger amounts of feces. In addition, the periparturient rise in cyst excretion observed in cattle, sheep, and goats would indicate that *G duodenalis* infection is maintained, although perhaps at a low level, in adult ruminants. It is not understood why *G duodenalis* infections in ruminants are chronic. Studies demonstrate that infected calves and lambs exhibit an extremely weak serologic immune response to *Giardia*, and this may account for the chronicity of infection [19,23]. Other parasite factors, such as the expression of antigenic variation, may also be contributing factors.

Clinical signs, pathology, pathogenesis

Diarrhea is the primary clinical sign associated with giardiasis in humans and companion animals. However, the importance of giardiasis as a cause of diarrhea in ruminants is still unclear. A number of studies have implicated

G duodenalis as the cause of diarrhea in ruminants [5,8,24], whereas others have found *G duodenalis* infections in ruminants not to be associated with diarrhea [25,26]. Because the vast majority of studies examining the clinical significance of *Giardia* in ruminants have been conducted in the field and not as controlled experiments, it is difficult to determine whether *G duodenalis* infections in ruminants result in clinical signs. The presence of *Giardia* cysts in diarrheic feces does not provide enough evidence to conclude that giardiasis is a cause of diarrhea in ruminants; diarrhea in ruminants is often multifactorial, with more than one pathogen detected. *G duodenalis* and *C parvum* may be found together in calves with diarrhea [5,24,25], and coinfection with *G duodenalis* and viral pathogens has also been reported [5,8,25]. The interaction between *G duodenalis* and other pathogens during the occurrence of diarrhea in ruminants has yet to be studied. A few experimental infections have demonstrated that *G duodenalis* has some capacity to cause noticeable clinical signs in ruminants. Experimental infection in goats resulted in decreased appetite, formless feces, and depression [18], whereas experimentally infected specific pathogen–free (SPF) lambs produced abnormal feces [20]. However, infection with *G duodenalis* on its own does not cause a severe or watery diarrhea in ruminants.

Although the clinical signs associated with giardiasis in ruminants appear to be mild, it should be emphasized that the presence or absence of clinical signs does not necessarily amount to the presence or absence of disease. A number of studies indicate that *G duodenalis* infections in ruminants result in pathogenic changes to the intestine, similar to those reported in infected humans and laboratory animals. In goats, villus blunting and crypt hyperplasia were observed in both the duodenum and jejunum following *G duodenalis* infection [18]. In calves, villus atrophy and an increase in the number of intraepithelial lymphocytes within the jejunum were also observed [27]. Even more striking was the observation that an increased brush border surface area and greater intestinal disaccharidase activity in the small intestine resulted from the elimination of *G duodenalis* infection in calves through drug therapy [2]. These pathologic changes mimic those observed in laboratory animals, which result in significant malabsorption [28,29]. Considering the chronicity of the infection, these pathologic changes have the potential to translate into significant losses with respect to ruminant production.

Impact on production

Unfortunately, little research has been conducted to determine whether giardiasis is a production-limiting disease of ruminants. Because the parasite is highly prevalent in ruminants, *G duodenalis*–free herds are virtually impossible to find. As a result, studies comparing milk production or growth rates between infected and noninfected herds cannot be performed. However, a well-controlled experiment using SPF lambs demonstrated that *G duodenalis* infections can have a significant impact on growth and performance [20]. In cattle, studies have attempted to examine the production impact of *G duodenalis* by treating calves with fenbendazole to eliminate the infection [30]. However, reinfection occurs rapidly after treatment, so no useful data could be provided on the potential production impact of this parasite.

Zoonotic potential and public health

Despite some concern about the role of ruminants as reservoirs for human infection, there are no reports of ruminants' causing giardiasis in humans, either through direct contact or through waterborne transmission. In addition, research employing molecular techniques has demonstrated that the species *G duodenalis* is composed of at least five distinct genetic groupings [31]. A number of these genetic groupings are believed to be host specific and of little concern with regard to zoonotic transmission. Recent studies indicate that at least 80% of *G duodenalis* infections in dairy cattle [21,32], 66% of infections in sheep [33], and 98% of infections in beef calves on range [34] are the result of *G duodenalis* corresponding to the livestock-specific Assemblage E genotype. Nevertheless, a portion of *G duodenalis* infections in ruminants are the result of *G duodenalis* corresponding to the zoonotic Assemblage A. Hence ruminants may pose some risk for transmission of the parasite to humans, but this risk appears minimal. Furthermore, it must be considered that the presence of Assemblage A in ruminants may be the result of human transmission or contamination; a previous study suggested that humans may be a source of *G duodenalis* infection for both cattle and wildlife [35]. Still, proper management of ruminant fecal waste must always be emphasized, because it may contain other pathogens and environmental contaminants.

Diagnosis

The observation of *Giardia* cysts in a fecal specimen by light microscopy remains a practical and inexpensive method of diagnosing giardiasis in ruminants. Generally, a flotation procedure using either zinc sulfate or sugar solution is recommended to concentrate cysts from a fecal specimen before microscopy, and centrifugation procedures are superior to bench-top methods [36]. Sodium nitrate, in the authors' experience, is not a good solution for detecting *Giardia* cysts. The zinc sulfate centrifugation/flotation technique is the best standard method for detecting *Giardia* cysts from a fecal sample. However, sugar flotation works adequately and is usually used in ruminant samples, because oocysts of *Eimeria* and *Cryptosporidium* may also be encountered. *Giardia* cysts are ovoid, measuring 8 to 15 μm in length and 7 to 10 μm in width. The cysts are somewhat transparent when viewed under the microscope; when floated using zinc sulfate, the interior of the cyst may collapse, resulting in the appearance of a crescent-shaped body at one end (Fig. 3). With practice, cysts may easily be visualized at 100× magnification, and confirmation is easily made at 400× magnification. The use of a calibrated ocular micrometer is highly recommended (for all parasitology diagnostics). It is important to ensure that the iris diaphragm of the microscope is reduced sufficiently before viewing a specimen prepared by flotation, to improve the visualization of *Giardia* cysts.

A number of other methods have been developed for the diagnosis of *G duodenalis* infection. Numerous immunoassay kits (ELISAs) are available that detect *G duodenalis* infection by means of coproantigens [37]. These tests have been widely adopted in the small animal clinic and diagnostic laboratory and should work adequately for ruminants, although studies need to confirm this. Immunofluorescence microscopy and polymerase chain reaction (PCR) diagnostic assays have also been developed to detect *G duodenalis* infections in ruminants [38,39]. Although these tests may offer greater sensitivity than light microscopy, they are specific only for *Giardia* and may not be practical for routine diagnostic parasitology where the ability to detect multiple parasites is required. In addition, immunofluorescence microscopy and PCR are costly and require specialized equipment. Thus, they tend to be restricted to the research or specialized diagnostic laboratory.

Control and treatment

No drug is currently licensed for treating giardiasis in ruminants, and whether *G duodenalis* infections in ruminants require treatment is debatable. Nevertheless, a number of studies have examined the efficacy of compounds

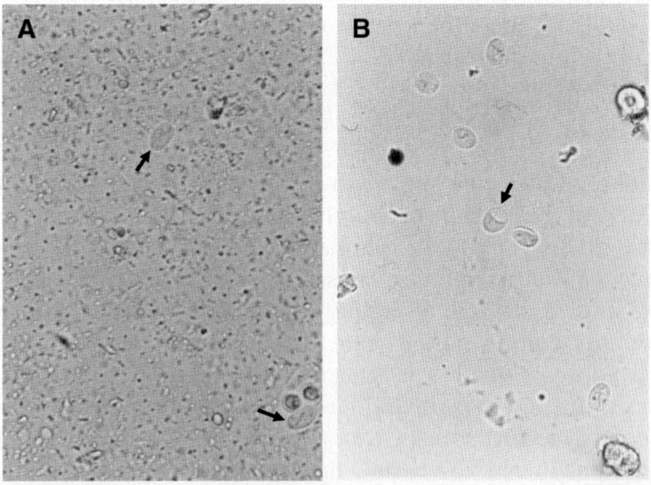

Fig. 3. Photomicrograph of *G duodenalis* cysts (*arrows*) from a direct smear (*A*) and after flotation using zinc sulfate (*B*). Cysts are approximately 10 μm in length. (*Courtesy of* Gary Conboy, DVM, Charlottetown, Prince Edward Island, Canada.)

for treating ruminants for giardiasis. The benzimidazoles, fenbendazole, and albendazole have significant efficacy against giardiasis in calves. Fenbendazole administered orally at 5 mg/kg per day for 3 days or 0.8 mg/kg per day for 6 days is efficacious in treating calves for giardiasis, as is albendazole at 20 mg/kg per day for 3 days [40,41]. In a recent study, paromomycin sulfate administered daily at 75 mg/kg for 5 days showed efficacy in eliminating *G duodenalis* infection from calves [42]. Unfortunately, treatment alone is insufficient for controlling *G duodenalis* infections in ruminants, because reinfection occurs rapidly [30,42]. Continual daily administration of a drug is likely to be required to keep ruminants free of the parasite, but such a treatment regimen is not practical.

No vaccine is available for the prevention and control of giardiasis in ruminants, although a vaccine is available for dogs [43]. Before work on the development of a vaccine for ruminants can take place, further research into the production impact and zoonotic potential of the parasite must be undertaken to determine whether vaccination is justified.

Minimizing the spread of *G duodenalis* infections among ruminants is difficult, and it is not possible to prevent infection from a practical standpoint. For example, in a well-managed dairy herd, calves housed individually became reinfected following treatment with fenbendazole, despite precautions taken by staff to prevent transmission and the extensive use of a disinfectant [30]. The low infectious dose and chronicity of infection result in most, if not all, ruminants' becoming infected. It is not known whether the infectious dose is related to the development (or severity) of clinical signs, so it may be useful to reduce exposure to cysts. Good husbandry, including prompt removal of feces from animal housing, regular cleaning and disinfecting of stalls, and ensuring adequate transfer of passive immunity, is likely to be beneficial in minimizing the potential impact of giardiasis on ruminants.

Cryptosporidiosis

Intestinal cryptosporidiosis due to infection with *C parvum* is a well-recognized cause of diarrhea in neonatal ruminants and has been reviewed extensively by others [44–47]. In ruminants, three species of *Cryptosporidium* are now recognized as common causes of infection. *C parvum* is the most extensively studied of these three species and is primarily a parasite of neonatal ruminants, colonizing the ileum and proximal portions of the large intestine. *C andersoni*, which was referred to as *C muris* in cattle before 2000 [48], resides in the abomasum and has so far only been identified in mature cattle. Recently, a third species, *C bovis*, which is morphologically identical to *C parvum* but infects calves at 2 to 7 months of age, has been proposed [49]. This species was previously referred to as the *Cryptosporidium* bovine B genotype. Of these three species, only *C parvum* is considered zoonotic, having been identified as a cause of gastrointestinal disease in humans.

Life cycle and transmission

The life cycle of *Cryptosporidium* is complex, involving both asexual and sexual reproductive stages (Fig. 4). Generally speaking, the life cycle is similar to that of the enteric coccidia, such as *Eimeria*, except that *Cryptosporidium* oocysts are passed fully sporulated from the host, and autoinfection may occur. In ruminants, following ingestion of the infective oocysts, sporozoites are released. In the case of *C parvum*, they invade the intestinal epithelium, whereas *C andersoni* colonizes the abomasum. The parasite undergoes development within the apical portion of the epithelial cell; although intracellular, *Cryptosporidium* does not develop within the host cell cytoplasm. Following the infection of the host cell, the parasite transforms into a circular trophozoite, which then undergoes asexual reproduction, becoming a meront. Merozoites within the meront are released from the epithelial cell and subsequently invade additional epithelial cells, where this asexual reproduction is repeated. Two types of *Cryptosporidium* meronts are produced. Type I meronts release merozoites that produce additional Type I meronts. However, some merozoites produce Type II meronts, which differentiate into macrogamonts and microgamonts. Microgametes released by microgamonts fertilize the macrogamont to form a zygote. This becomes an oocyst following the formation of a resistant oocyst wall and after it has undergone sporogony to produce four sporozoites within the oocyst. Thick- and thin-walled oocysts are formed by *Cryptosporidium*. The thick-walled oocysts are environmentally resistant and are passed in the feces of the host. Thin-walled oocysts rupture in the intestine of the host and are believed to be important as a vehicle for autoinfection.

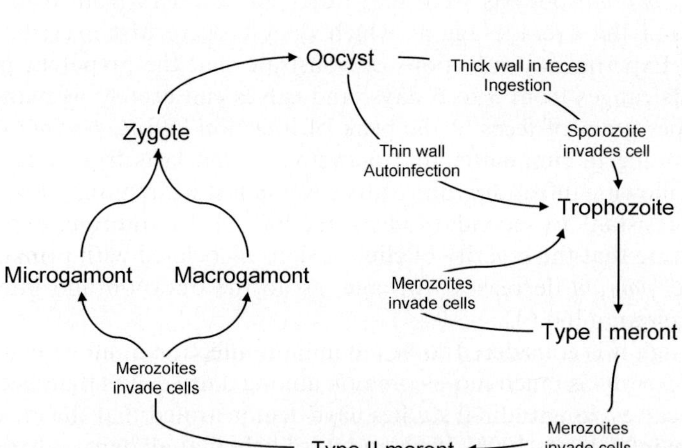

Fig. 4. Life cycle of *Cryptosporidium* spp. *C parvum* invades epithelial cells primarily in the distal small intestine, but it can also be found in the proximal small intestine and colon. *C andersoni* resides in the gastric glands of the abomasum. The role of recently discovered gregarine-like extracellular stages in the life cycle is not known.

Cryptosporidium oocysts are immediately infective once they exit the host, and young ruminants can excrete more than 10^7 *Cryptosporidium* oocysts per gram of feces [45,46]. Direct transmission via the fecal–oral route is the most common and important route for the parasite, and the minimum infectious dose for *C parvum* is 30 oocysts [50]. Transmission is aided by the extremely resistant nature of the oocysts in the environment: they can remain infectious for months in cool, moist conditions. *Cryptosporidium* oocysts are also resistant to standard levels of chlorination [4]. As a result, epidemic outbreaks of cryptosporidiosis in the human population are often associated with waterborne transmission [51]. However, the role of ruminants in these waterborne epidemics is not clear (see further discussion).

Recently, novel extracellular stages of *C parvum* and *C andersoni* have been identified following in vitro culture of the parasites [52,53]. These extracellular stages resemble stages from the gregarine parasites, providing evidence that *Cryptosporidium* may not be a coccidian. However, the role of these stages in the in vivo life cycle of the parasite or the environment is not understood at this time.

Epidemiology

C parvum is recognized as one of the most common infectious causes of intestinal disease in neonatal calves, lambs, and kids [45–47], and infections have been reported in elk [14,54], deer [55], and water buffalo [56]. *C parvum* infections have been observed in ruminants as young as 3 days but are most common in ruminants from 1 to 3 weeks of age [45,46]; infections are rare in calves older than 30 days [57,58]. In a longitudinal study examining dairy calves, *C parvum* oocysts were first observed in calves from 6 to 42 days of age, and the average age at which oocysts were first excreted was 16 days [5]. Experimental infections demonstrate that the prepatent period in ruminants ranges from 3 to 6 days, and calves can excrete as many as 10^7 oocysts per gram of feces at the peak of infection [59]. *C parvum* infection is self-limiting in ruminants, and oocyst excretion lasts from 1 to 2 weeks [5,59]. Following infection, ruminants develop lasting immunity to *C parvum* and are resistant to secondary challenge [60,61]. In addition, experiments demonstrate that the severity of clinical signs associated with primary exposure to *C parvum* decreases with age, as do the duration and intensity of oocyst excretion [60,61].

Although it is considered to be a common infection in all neonatal ruminants, *C parvum* is much more common among dairy calves than beef calves. In dairy calves, longitudinal studies have demonstrated that the incidence of *C parvum* infection is 100% [5,6], and it is likely that all dairy calves become infected with *C parvum* in the first few weeks of life [47]. However, the epidemiology of *C parvum* in beef calves appears to be quite different. In a recent study, *C parvum* was detected in only 3% of calves from cow-calf operations in western Canada [62]. A longitudinal study from the same region revealed an incidence of only 5% in beef calves [15]. In the United States, reported prevalence of *C parvum* in cow-calf operations ranges from 0% to 13%, with an overall prevalence in calves of 5.6% [63]. It would appear logical that the reduced stocking density associated with the cow-calf operations typical of western North America accounts for the lower prevalence of *C parvum* infection, and evidence supports this theory [64,65]. However, recent studies from Europe indicate that the prevalence of *C parvum* in beef calves is significantly lower than that in dairy calves when housed in similar conditions [66], and in a recent study the incidence of *C parvum* infection in confined and semiconfined beef calves did not exceed 25% [65]. These results would indicate that factors other than confinement influence the prevalence and infection patterns of *C parvum* in calves.

C andersoni infections were first reported in cattle in 1987 (when it was called *C muris*) [67]. Since then, infections have been reported in cattle throughout the world [68]. *C andersoni* appears to be limited to cattle: experimental attempts to infect lambs and goats have failed [69,70]. In a recent survey, however, *C andersoni* was detected in the feces of a single sheep [33]. The overall prevalence of *C andersoni* appears to be low, ranging from 2% to 5% [58,71,72], although prevalences of 30% to 40% have been reported in some herds [15,66,71]. *C andersoni* infections primarily occur in post-weaned beef and dairy cattle, as well as in mature cattle [15,57,58]. In contrast to *C parvum* infections, *C andersoni* infections are chronic in cattle and may persist for months or even years [47,68].

Little is known about the newly proposed species *C bovis*. It appears to be common among older calves [49,58] and may have been confused with *C parvum* in previous studies, because they are morphologically identical.

Clinical signs, pathology, pathogenesis

C parvum is a well-known cause of diarrhea in neonatal ruminants. Numerous reports detail the occurrence of clinical disease due to cryptosporidiosis in calves, lambs, goat kids, and other ruminants [45,46]. The clinical signs of cryptosporidiosis are similar in calves, sheep, and kids and include diarrhea, which is often pale yellow with mucus, lethargy, anorexia, and dehydration [45,46,59,73]. The clinical signs become evident 3 to 5 days following infection, and their duration can vary from 4 to 18 days. Severe cryptosporidiosis can result in extreme dehydration, metabolic acidosis, and death, but these cases are rare. Although it is less frequently identified in beef calves than in dairy calves, outbreaks of cryptosporidiosis can be more severe in beef calves than in dairy calves and may result in mortality as high as 30% [68]. In many of these cases, the introduction of dairy calves into the herd during calving season was a contributing factor. In addition, low levels of serum selenium in beef herds were associated with high mortality due to cryptosporidiosis [68]. It is important to emphasize that *C parvum* is commonly identified along with other enteropathogens during cases of neonatal diarrhea [46,47], and the parasite may often be identified in calves that have no signs of clinical disease [5,25]. The severity of cryptosporidiosis is influenced by a number of factors, including the infectious doses, herd immunity, presence of concurrent infections, nutrition, and husbandry [68]. Thus, in most well-managed herds, cryptosporidiosis due to *C parvum* is typically a mild disease and not a serious health concern [47].

The clinical signs associated with intestinal cryptosporidiosis are the result of both malabsorption and an increase in fluid secretion. Although the exact mechanisms are still not fully understood, both parasite and host factors play a role. *C parvum* primarily colonizes the distal small intestine (Fig. 5); however, the parasite may also infect the proximal small intestine, as well as the cecum and colon [74,75]. Infection results in villous atrophy, villous fusion, crypt hyperplasia, disruption of the intestinal microvilli, and the infiltration of inflammatory cells [73–75]. These changes can result in malabsorption through the loss of intestinal surface area, loss of membrane-bound intestinal enzymes, and impaired nutrient and electrolyte transport [76]. In addition, the presence of a cholera-like toxin, secreted by the parasite, may also be involved in the development of a secretory type of diarrhea [77]. Recent studies suggest that *Cryptosporidium* can also induce apoptosis [78,79] and disrupt the epithelial tight junction, resulting in the loss of barrier function [78]. The culmination of these pathologic changes is the development of both a malabsorptive and a secretory diarrhea.

Abomasal cryptosporidiosis, caused by *C andersoni*, does not result in the development of noticeable clinical signs. Nevertheless, the parasite affects the peptic and pyloric glands (Fig. 6), resulting in dilatation of the gastric gland, hypertrophy of the gastric mucosa, and hypertrophy of the epithelial lining [47,67,80]. It has been reported that abomasal cryptosporidiosis

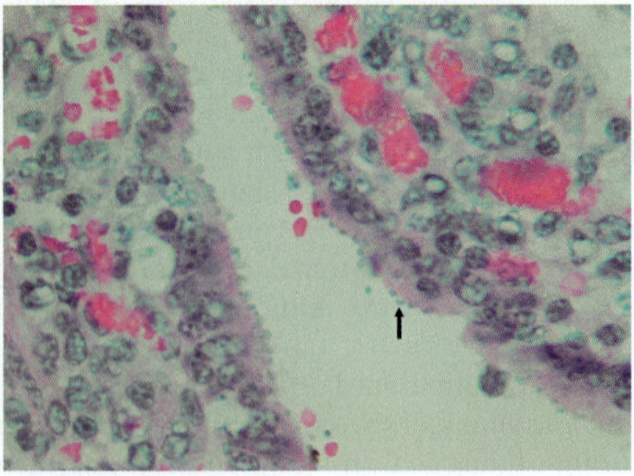

Fig. 5. Histologic section of small intestine of a 10-day-old calf (hematoxylin-eosin) showing various stages of *C parvum* in the epithelial brush border (*arrow*). (Original magnification ×100.) (*Courtesy of* Mandy O'Hara, BVMS, MACVSc, Perth, Australia.)

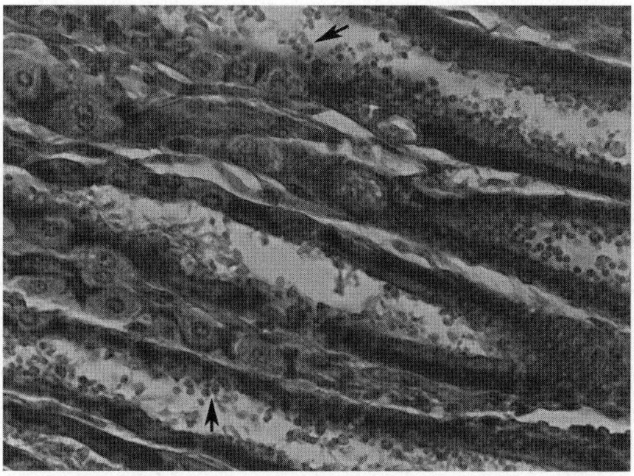

Fig. 6. Histologic section of abomasum from an 18-month-old feedlot steer (hematoxylin-eosin) showing numerous stages of *C andersoni* in the epithelium and lumen of the gastric glands (*arrows*).

somewhat resembles type 2 ostertagiasis, because an increase in abomasal pH and plasma pepsinogen levels are associated with the infection [47].

Impact on production

No evidence indicates that intestinal cryptosporidiosis results in any long-term production effects in ruminants. In studies where various drug therapies were employed to control cryptosporidiosis in ruminants, there were no differences between treated and untreated groups with respect to weight gain [81,82]. Hence the economic impact of *C parvum* infections in ruminants is limited to losses due to mortality and costs involved in treating animals for clinical signs. Nevertheless, these costs may be substantial in some outbreaks of cryptosporidiosis.

Abomasal cryptosporidiosis may be an important production-limiting disease of cattle. In fact, *C andersoni* infections were first discovered during an investigation of feedlot cattle that had a lower than expected daily weight gain [67]. A decreased feed efficiency has been reported in feedlot cattle with *C andersoni* infections [83]. Dairy cows excreting *C andersoni* oocysts in their feces were found to produce significantly less milk than cows in which oocysts could not be detected [84]. No reports on the effect of *C andersoni* on range cattle exist, and further studies are required to confirm these previous findings. However, the observations made so far indicate that *C andersoni* could be of economic importance to both the beef and dairy industries.

Zoonotic potential and public health significance

Ruminants, particularly cattle, are often considered reservoirs for outbreaks of cryptosporidiosis in humans. However, several outbreaks of human cryptosporidiosis that were initially attributed to agricultural runoff have now been shown to be of human origin. An example is the Milwaukee outbreak in which *C hominis*, not *C parvum,* was most likely responsible, indicating a human source of the contamination [85]. Cattle have not been conclusively identified as the source of any waterborne outbreak of cryptosporidiosis in North America, so it is likely that humans are the main source for human outbreaks of cryptosporidiosis.

C parvum is a zoonotic parasite, and numerous reports of cryptosporidiosis outbreaks in humans are associated with farm visits and contact with calves [86–88]. However, research into the epidemiology of *C parvum* infection, including recent research employing molecular techniques, indicates that only young ruminants, primarily neonates, pose a risk for the zoonotic transmission of *Cryptosporidium*. *C parvum* infections are rare in dairy calves older than 30 days, and infections in older calves and adult cattle are most commonly due to *C andersoni* and the recently proposed *C bovis*, which are not zoonotic [57]. In addition, older lambs and adult sheep are not infected with *C parvum* [33]. Recently, the human infectious *C hominis* was detected in 2 of 411 bovine fecal samples in the United Kingdom, but it is not known whether these were active infections. Given that neonatal ruminants, and dairy calves in particular, pose the greatest risk for direct or waterborne zoonotic transmission of *C parvum*, the risk may be readily managed. Surface and ground water should be protected from young ruminants and their feces, and such manure should be composted or spread on a field where runoff cannot occur. Composting generates sufficient heat to kill *Cryptosporidium*, and spreading of manure on fields enables UV light and desiccation to kill oocysts [89]. The manure of older ruminants, including cattle on range, is generally not a zoonotic concern with respect to *Cryptosporidium*.

Diagnosis

Intestinal cryptosporidiosis should be included in the differential diagnosis in all cases of neonatal diarrhea in ruminants. Abomasal cryptosporidiosis must also be considered in dairy and feedlot cattle that are not performing as expected. The standard method of diagnosing both *C parvum* and *C andersoni* infections remains the observation of oocysts in the feces (Fig. 7). Flotation with saturated sugar is generally the preferred method of concentrating *Cryptosporidium* oocysts. *C parvum* oocysts are round and measure 4 to 6 μm in diameter. *C andersoni* oocysts are ovoid and slightly larger than *C parvum* oocysts, measuring 6 to 8 μm in length by 5.0 to 6.5 μm in width. *Cryptosporidium* oocysts do not contain sporocysts. They often appear with a slight pink hue when floated in sucrose, and small dark granules may be seen within the oocysts. Because of their small size, oocysts are best observed at 400× magnification. The oocysts are quite buoyant and will be found high in the focal plane, just beneath the coverslip. As a result, other parasites, such as *Eimeria*, will appear slightly out of focus

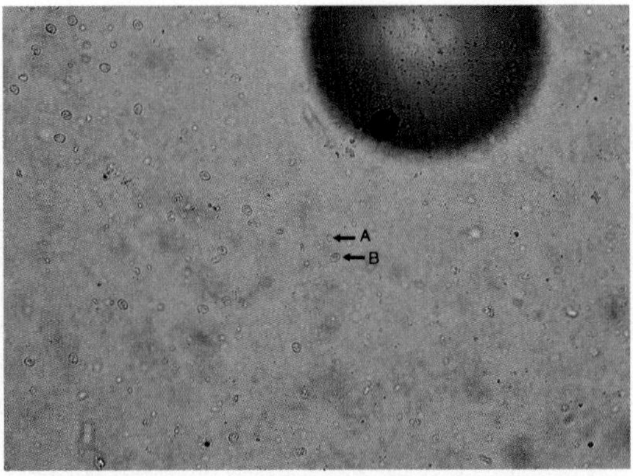

Fig. 7. Photomicrograph of sugar flotation of bovine feces seeded with *C parvum* oocysts (A) and *C andersoni* oocysts (B). (Original magnification ×400.) *C parvum* oocysts are approximately 5 μm in diameter. *C andersoni* oocysts are approximately 8 μm in length. Note that the background is out of focus as the oocysts float high in sugar solution.

when one is viewing *Cryptosporidium*. A number of staining techniques, such as acid-fast stains, have also been used to aid in detecting *Cryptosporidium* oocysts [90].

In addition to light microscopy–based procedures, a number of coproantigen-based immunoassay kits are available for diagnosing *C parvum* infections [37]. Although these tests should be effective in detecting *C parvum* infections, it is not known whether they may be used to detect *C andersoni* infections. Immunofluorescence microscopy and PCR-based diagnostic tests have also been developed and are widely used in research and in some specialist diagnostic laboratories [38,39]. As mentioned earlier, molecular and antibody-based diagnostic assays can be more sensitive than microscopy, but they can also be costly and will not detect other parasites that may be of importance.

Control and treatment

Currently, no drugs are licensed for treating cryptosporidiosis in ruminants in North America. Hence, in severe cases of neonatal cryptosporidiosis, supportive therapy through fluid replacement and treatment of metabolic acidosis with intravenous sodium bicarbonate solutions may be required.

In Europe, halofuginone lactate has been registered as a chemotherapeutic agent for treating cryptosporidiosis in cattle. Halofuginone lactate at 60 to 125 μg/kg per day can reduce the severity and incidence of diarrhea in calves and delay the onset of oocyst excretion, but it does not prevent excretion of oocysts [82,91,92]. However, toxic side effects of the drug were observed at 500 μg/kg/d [92]. Experimental trials have shown that paromomycin reduces oocyst excretion, as well as the frequency and duration of diarrhea, in calves and lambs [93–95]. In goats and kids, decoquinate has been shown to reduce the severity of cryptosporidiosis and oocyst excretion [96], but decoquinate did not have an effect on oocyst shedding or clinical signs in calves [97].

Numerous vaccination trials have been conducted in calves to control cryptosporidiosis [98]. Both active and passive immunization strategies have been employed, with some studies reporting a reduction in the severity of clinical signs and the number of oocysts excreted. However, vaccines have not been able to prevent infection. The need for a vaccine or a drug to control intestinal cryptosporidiosis in calves is debatable. The infection is self-limiting, ruminants develop immunity following initial infections, and, in most cases, clinical signs are mild. It should also be emphasized that a prophylactic approach to the use of chemotherapies has been employed in the majority of clinical trials. Because infections with *C parvum* do not affect production in ruminants over the long term, the costs associated with prophylactic chemotherapy or vaccination may not be justified.

Management strategies for controlling cryptosporidiosis in ruminants are similar to those that are employed to control coccidiosis. The use of good husbandry—isolation of animals with diarrhea, cleaning of stalls before the introduction of calves, prompt removal and disposal of feces, and ensuring that calves receive adequate colostrum—can reduce the number of oocysts animals are exposed to and increase the resistance of calves to *C parvum* and other enteropathogens [99]. In addition, dairy calves should not be introduced to beef herds during calving season. Completely preventing exposure of young ruminants to *C parvum* oocysts is not possible, because oocysts are resistant to most commercial disinfectants, unless they are used at concentrations that make them hazardous [99]. It must be emphasized that *C parvum* is a zoonotic parasite, so good hygiene, especially frequent and thorough hand washing, must be practiced by those who work with or handle young ruminants.

Currently, there are no investigations into chemotherapies or vaccines to control abomasal cryptosporidiosis. Although abomasal cryptosporidiosis does not appear to be a severe disease of cattle, research into the control of *C andersoni* is warranted by its potential production impact on feedlot and dairy cattle.

Summary

G duodenalis is one of the most common parasites found in ruminants. Most if not all ruminants become infected with *G duodenalis* at some point in their first few months of life. Giardiasis is chronic in ruminants, and, although it does not result in severe clinical signs, it does cause intestinal pathologic conditions that may result in malabsorption. Thus, giardiasis may be a production-limiting disease of ruminants. Studies employing molecular techniques demonstrate that the vast majority of ruminants are infected by a livestock-specific genotype of *G duodenalis*. Hence, although ruminants may serve as a potential reservoir for giardiasis in humans, they pose much less of a risk than was previously thought.

C parvum remains an important cause of diarrhea in neonatal ruminants. Still, no treatment exists for cryptosporidiosis in North America. Recent research indicates that the parasite is much more common and important in dairy calves than in beef calves, and only young ruminants, generally less than 1 month of age, are infected with *C parvum*. Thus the zoonotic risk associated with *C parvum* infections in ruminants is limited to young animals and is easily managed. Less understood than intestinal cryptosporidiosis, abomasal cryptosporidiosis, caused by *C andersoni*, is an emerging disease in cattle that may have a significant impact on production in both beef and dairy cattle. In general, *C andersoni* infections are not common in cattle, but the prevalence can be high in some herds, and infections last months or even years. Further research is required if we are better to understand the significance of abomasal cryptosporidiosis.

References

[1] Thompson RC. The zoonotic significance and molecular epidemiology of *Giardia* and giardiasis. Vet Parasitol 2004;126:15–35.

[2] O'Handley RM, Buret AG, McAllister TA, et al. Giardiasis in dairy calves: effects of fenbendazole treatment on intestinal structure and function. Int J Parasitol 2001;31:73–9.

[3] Rendtorff RC. The experimental transmission of human intestinal protozoan parasites. II. Giardia lamblia cysts given in capsules. Am J Hyg 1954;59:209–20.

[4] Betancourt WQ, Rose JB. Drinking water treatment processes for removal of *Cryptosporidium* and *Giardia*. Vet Parasitol 2004;126:219–34.

[5] O'Handley RM, Cockwill C, McAllister TA, et al. Duration of naturally acquired giardiosis and cryptosporidiosis in dairy calves and their association with diarrhea. J Am Vet Med Assoc 1999;214:391–6.

[6] Xiao L, Herd RP. Infection pattern of *Cryptosporidium* and *Giardia* in calves. Vet Parasitol 1994;55:257–62.

[7] McDonough SP, Stull CL, Osburn BI. Enteric pathogens in intensively reared veal calves. Am J Vet Res 1994;55:1516–20.

[8] St. Jean G, Couture Y, Dubreuil P, et al. Diagnosis of Giardia infection in 14 calves. J Am Vet Med Assoc 1987;191:831–2.

[9] Taylor MA, Catchpole J, Marshall RN, et al. Giardiasis in lambs at pasture. Vet Rec 1993; 133:131–3.

[10] Buret A, denHollander N, Wallis PM, et al. Zoonotic potential of giardiasis in domestic ruminants. J Infect Dis 1990;162:231–7.

[11] Bomfim TC, Huber F, Gomes RS, et al. Natural infection by *Giardia* sp. and *Cryptosporidium* sp. in dairy goats, associated with possible risk factors of the studied properties. Vet Parasitol 2005;134:9–13.

[12] Castro-Hermida JA, Delafosse A, Pors I, et al. Giardia duodenalis and Cryptosporidium parvum infections in adult goats and their implications for neonatal kids. Vet Rec 2005; 157:623–7.

[13] Al-Jabr OA, Mohammed GE, Al-Hamdan BA. Giardiosis in camels (Camelus dromedarius). Vet Rec 2005;157:350–2.

[14] Deng MQ, Cliver DO. Improved immunofluorescence assay for detection of *Giardia* and *Cryptosporidium* from asymptomatic adult cervine animals. Parasitol Res 1999;85:733–6.

[15] Ralston BJ, McAllister TA, Olson ME. Prevalence and infection pattern of naturally acquired giardiasis and cryptosporidiosis in range beef calves and their dams. Vet Parasitol 2003;114:113–22.
[16] Xiao L, Herd RP, McClure KE. Periparturient rise in the excretion of *Giardia* sp. cysts and *Cryptosporidium parvum* oocysts as a source of infection for lambs. J Parasitol 1994;80:55–9.
[17] Taminelli V, Eckert J, Sydler T, et al. Experimental infection of calves and sheep with bovine *Giardia* isolates. Schweiz Arch Tierheilkd 1989;131:551–64 [in German].
[18] Koudela B, Vitovec J. Experimental giardiasis in goat kids. Vet Parasitol 1998;74:9–18.
[19] O'Handley RM, Ceri H, Anette C, et al. Passive immunity and serological immune response in dairy calves associated with natural *Giardia duodenalis* infections. Vet Parasitol 2003;113: 89–98.
[20] Olson ME, McAllister TA, Deselliers L, et al. Effects of giardiasis on production in a domestic ruminant (lamb) model. Am J Vet Res 1995;56:1470–4.
[21] Trout JM, Santin M, Greiner E, et al. Prevalence and genotypes of *Giardia duodenalis* in post-weaned dairy calves. Vet Parasitol 2005;130:177–83.
[22] Uehlinger FD, Barkema HW, Dixon BR, et al. Dynamics and zoonotic potential of *Giardia duodenalis* and *Cryptosporidium* spp. in a veterinary college teaching herd. Paper presented at the 20th International Conference of the World Association for the Advancement of Veterinary Parasitology. Christchurch, New Zealand, October 16–20, 2005.
[23] Yanke SJ, Ceri H, McAllister TA, et al. Serum immune response to *Giardia duodenalis* in experimentally infected lambs. Vet Parasitol 1998;75:9–19.
[24] Xiao L, Herd RP, Rings DM. Concurrent infections of *Giardia* and *Cryptosporidium* on two Ohio farms with calf diarrhea. Vet Parasitol 1993;51:41–8.
[25] Bjorkman C, Svensson C, Christensson B, et al. *Cryptosporidium parvum* and *Giardia intestinalis* in calf diarrhoea in Sweden. Acta Vet Scand 2003;44:145–52.
[26] Huetink RE, van der Giessen JW, Noordhuizen JP, et al. Epidemiology of *Cryptosporidium* spp. and *Giardia duodenalis* on a dairy farm. Vet Parasitol 2001;102:53–67.
[27] Ruest N, Couture Y, Faubert GM, et al. Morphological changes in the jejunum of calves naturally infected with *Giardia* spp. and *Cryptosporidium* spp. Vet Parasitol 1997;69:177–86.
[28] Buret A, Gall DG, Olson ME. Effects of murine giardiasis on growth, intestinal morphology, and disaccharidase activity. J Parasitol 1990;76:403–9.
[29] Buret A, Hardin JA, Olson ME, et al. Pathophysiology of small intestinal malabsorption in gerbils infected with *Giardia lamblia*. Gastroenterology 1992;103:506–13.
[30] O'Handley RM, Cockwill C, Jelinski M, et al. Effects of repeat fenbendazole treatment in dairy calves with giardiosis on cyst excretion, clinical signs and production. Vet Parasitol 2000;89:209–18.
[31] Hunter PR, Thompson RC. The zoonotic transmission of *Giardia* and *Cryptosporidium*. Int J Parasitol 2005;35:1181–90.
[32] O'Handley RM, Olson ME, Fraser D, et al. Prevalence and genotypic characterisation of *Giardia* in dairy calves from Western Australia and Western Canada. Vet Parasitol 2000; 90:193–200.
[33] Ryan UM, Bath C, Robertson I, et al. Sheep may not be an important zoonotic reservoir for *Cryptosporidium* and *Giardia* parasites. Appl Environ Microbiol 2005;71:4992–7.
[34] Appelbee AJ, Frederick LM, Heitman TL, et al. Prevalence and genotyping of *Giardia duodenalis* from beef calves in Alberta, Canada. Vet Parasitol 2003;112:289–94.
[35] Graczyk TK, Bosco-Nizeyi J, Ssebide B, et al. Anthropozoonotic *Giardia duodenalis* genotype (Assemblage) A infections in habitats of free-ranging human-habituated gorillas, Uganda. J Parasitol 2002;88:905–9.
[36] Zajac AM, Johnson J, King SE. Evaluation of the importance of centrifugation as a component of zinc sulfate fecal flotation examinations. J Am Anim Hosp Assoc 2002;38:221–4.
[37] Garcia LS, Shimizu RY. Evaluation of nine immunoassay kits (enzyme immunoassay and direct fluorescence) for detection of *Giardia lamblia* and *Cryptosporidium parvum* in human fecal specimens. J Clin Microbiol 1997;35:1526–9.

[38] Xiao L, Herd RP. Quantitation of *Giardia* cysts and *Cryptosporidium* oocysts in fecal samples by direct immunofluorescence assay. J Clin Microbiol 1993;31:2944–6.
[39] Morgan UM, Thompson RC. Molecular detection of parasitic protozoa. Parasitology 1998; 117(Suppl):S73–85.
[40] O'Handley RM, Olson ME, McAllister TA, et al. Efficacy of fenbendazole for treatment of giardiasis in calves. Am J Vet Res 1997;58:384–8.
[41] Xiao L, Saeed K, Herd RP. Efficacy of albendazole and fenbendazole against *Giardia* infection in cattle. Vet Parasitol 1996;61:165–70.
[42] Geurden T, Claerebout E, Dursin L, et al. The efficacy of an oral treatment with paromomycin against an experimental infection with *Giardia* in calves. Vet Parasitol 2006;135:241–7.
[43] Olson ME, Ceri H, Morck DW. *Giardia* vaccination. Parasitol Today 2000;16:213–7.
[44] Kirkpatrick CE. Cryptosporidium infection as a cause of calf diarrhea. Vet Clin North Am Food Anim Pract 1985;1:515–28.
[45] Fayer R, Speer CA, Dubey JP. The general biology of *Cryptosporidium*. In: Fayer R, editor. *Cryptosporidium* and cryptosporidiosis. Boca Raton (FL): CRC Press; 1997. p. 1–33.
[46] de Graaf DC, Vanopdenbosch E, Ortega-Mora LM, et al. A review of the importance of cryptosporidiosis in farm animals. Int J Parasitol 1999;29:1269–87.
[47] Anderson BC. Cryptosporidiosis in bovine and human health. J Dairy Sci 1998;81:3036–41.
[48] Lindsay DS, Upton SJ, Owens DS, et al. *Cryptosporidium andersoni* n. sp. (Apicomplexa: Cryptosporiidae) from cattle, Bos taurus. J Eukaryot Microbiol 2000;47:91–5.
[49] Fayer R, Santin M, Xiao L. *Cryptosporidium bovis* n. sp. (Apicomplexa: Cryptosporidiidae) in cattle (Bos taurus). J Parasitol 2005;91:624–9.
[50] DuPont HL, Chappell CL, Sterling CR, et al. The infectivity of *Cryptosporidium parvum* in healthy volunteers. N Engl J Med 1995;332:855–9.
[51] Mac Kenzie WR, Hoxie NJ, Proctor ME, et al. A massive outbreak in Milwaukee of *Cryptosporidium* infection transmitted through the public water supply. N Engl J Med 1994;331: 161–7.
[52] Hijjawi NS, Meloni BP, Ryan UM, et al. Successful in vitro cultivation of *Cryptosporidium andersoni*: evidence for the existence of novel extracellular stages in the life cycle and implications for the classification of *Cryptosporidium*. Int J Parasitol 2002;32:1719–26.
[53] Hijjawi NS, Meloni BP, Ng'anzo M, et al. Complete development of *Cryptosporidium parvum* in host cell–free culture. Int J Parasitol 2004;34:769–77.
[54] Pople NC, Allen AL, Woodbury MR. A retrospective study of neonatal mortality in farmed elk. Can Vet J 2001;42:925–8.
[55] Tzipori S, Angus KW, Campbell I, et al. Diarrhea in young red deer associated with infection with *Cryptosporidium*. J Infect Dis 1981;144:170–5.
[56] Gomez-Couso H, Amar CF, McLauchlin J, et al. Characterisation of a *Cryptosporidium* isolate from water buffalo (*Bubalus bubalis*) by sequencing of a fragment of the *Cryptosporidium* oocyst wall protein gene (COWP). Vet Parasitol 2005;131:139–44.
[57] Fayer R, Santin M, Trout JM, et al. Prevalence of species and genotypes of *Cryptosporidium* found in 1–2-year-old dairy cattle in the eastern United States. Vet Parasitol 2006;135: 105–12.
[58] Santin M, Trout JM, Xiao L, et al. Prevalence and age-related variation of *Cryptosporidium* species and genotypes in dairy calves. Vet Parasitol 2004;122:103–17.
[59] Fayer R, Gasbarre L, Pasquali P, et al. *Cryptosporidium parvum* infection in bovine neonates: dynamic clinical, parasitic and immunologic patterns. Int J Parasitol 1998;28:49–56.
[60] Harp JA, Woodmansee DB, Moon HW. Resistance of calves to Cryptosporidium parvum: effects of age and previous exposure. Infect Immun 1990;58:2237–40.
[61] Ortega-Mora LM, Wright SE. Age-related resistance in ovine cryptosporidiosis: patterns of infection and humoral immune response. Infect Immun 1994;62:5003–9.
[62] Gow S, Waldner C. An examination of the prevalence of and risk factors for shedding of *Cryptosporidium* spp. and *Giardia* spp. in cows and calves from western Canadian cow-calf herds. Vet Parasitol 2006;137:50–61.

[63] Atwill ER, Johnson E, Klingborg DJ, et al. Age, geographic, and temporal distribution of fecal shedding of *Cryptosporidium parvum* oocysts in cow-calf herds. Am J Vet Res 1999; 60:420–5.

[64] Atwill ER, Johnson EM, Pereira MG. Association of herd composition, stocking rate, and duration of calving season with fecal shedding of *Cryptosporidium parvum* oocysts in beef herds. J Am Vet Med Assoc 1999;215:1833–8.

[65] Jager M, Gauly M, Bauer C, et al. Endoparasites in calves of beef cattle herds: management systems dependent and genetic influences. Vet Parasitol 2005;131:173–91.

[66] Kvac M, Kouba M, Vitovec J. Age-related and housing-dependence of *Cryptosporidium* infection of calves from dairy and beef herds in South Bohemia, Czech Republic. Vet Parasitol 2006;137:202–9.

[67] Anderson BC. Abomasal cryptosporidiosis in cattle. Vet Pathol 1987;24:235–8.

[68] Olson ME, O'Handley RM, Ralston BJ, et al. Update on *Cryptosporidium* and *Giardia* infections in cattle. Trends Parasitol 2004;20:185–91.

[69] Kvac M, Ditrich O, Kouba M, et al. Failed attempt of *Cryptosporidium andersoni* infection in lambs. Folia Parasitol (Praha) 2004;51:373–4.

[70] Koudela B, Modry D, Vitovec J. Infectivity of *Cryptosporidium muris* isolated from cattle. Vet Parasitol 1998;76:181–8.

[71] Anderson BC. Prevalence of *Cryptosporidium muris*–like oocysts among cattle populations of the United States: preliminary report. J Protozool 1991;38:14S–5S.

[72] Olson ME, Guselle NJ, O'Handley RM, et al. *Giardia* and *Cryptosporidium* in dairy calves in British Columbia. Can Vet J 1997;38:703–6.

[73] Koudela B, Jiri V. Experimental cryptosporidiosis in kids. Vet Parasitol 1997;71:273–81.

[74] Angus KW, Tzipori S, Gray EW. Intestinal lesions in specific-pathogen-free lambs associated with a cryptosporidium from calves with diarrhea. Vet Pathol 1982;19:67–78.

[75] Heine J, Pohlenz JF, Moon HW, et al. Enteric lesions and diarrhea in gnotobiotic calves monoinfected with *Cryptosporidium* species. J Infect Dis 1984;150:768–75.

[76] Thompson RC, Olson ME, Zhu G, et al. *Cryptosporidium* and cryptosporidiosis. Adv Parasitol 2005;59:77–158.

[77] Guarino A, Canani RB, Pozio E, et al. Enterotoxic effect of stool supernatant of *Cryptosporidium*-infected calves on human jejunum. Gastroenterology 1994;106:28–34.

[78] Buret AG, Chin AC, Scott KG. Infection of human and bovine epithelial cells with *Cryptosporidium andersoni* induces apoptosis and disrupts tight junctional ZO-1: effects of epidermal growth factor. Int J Parasitol 2003;33:1363–71.

[79] Mele R, Gomez Morales MA, Tosini F, et al. *Cryptosporidium parvum* at different developmental stages modulates host cell apoptosis in vitro. Infect Immun 2004;72:6061–7.

[80] Kvac M, Vitovec J. Prevalence and pathogenicity of *Cryptosporidium andersoni* in one herd of beef cattle. J Vet Med B Infect Dis Vet Public Health 2003;50:451–7.

[81] Castro-Hermida JA, Pors I, Otero-Espinar F, et al. Efficacy of alpha-cyclodextrin against experimental cryptosporidiosis in neonatal goats. Vet Parasitol 2004;120:35–41.

[82] Jarvie BD, Trotz-Williams LA, McKnight DR, et al. Effect of halofuginone lactate on the occurrence of Cryptosporidium parvum and growth of neonatal dairy calves. J Dairy Sci 2005;88:1801–6.

[83] Ralston BJ, Cockwill C, Guselle NJ, et al. Prevalence of *Giardia* and *Cryptosporidium andersoni* and their effects on performance in feedlot beef cattle. Canadian Journal of Animal Science 2003;83:153–9.

[84] Esteban E, Anderson BC. *Cryptosporidium muris*: prevalence, persistency, and detrimental effect on milk production in a drylot dairy. J Dairy Sci 1995;78:1068–72.

[85] Zhou L, Singh A, Jiang J, et al. Molecular surveillance of Cryptosporidium spp. in raw wastewater in Milwaukee: implications for understanding outbreak occurrence and transmission dynamics. J Clin Microbiol 2003;41:5254–7.

[86] Smith KE, Stenzel SA, Bender JB, et al. Outbreaks of enteric infections caused by multiple pathogens associated with calves at a farm day camp. Pediatr Infect Dis J 2004;23:1098–104.

[87] Preiser G, Preiser L, Madeo L. An outbreak of cryptosporidiosis among veterinary science students who work with calves. J Am Coll Health 2003;51:213–5.
[88] Miron D, Kenes J, Dagan R. Calves as a source of an outbreak of cryptosporidiosis among young children in an agricultural closed community. Pediatr Infect Dis J 1991;10:438–41.
[89] Van Herk FH, McAllister TA, Cockwill C, et al. Inactivation of *Giardia* cysts and *Cryptosporidium* oocysts in beef feedlot manure by thermophilic windrow composting. Compost Sci Util 2004;12:235–41.
[90] Garcia LS, Bruckner DA, Brewer TC, et al. Techniques for the recovery and identification of *Cryptosporidium* oocysts from stool specimens. J Clin Microbiol 1983;18:185–90.
[91] Naciri M, Mancassola R, Yvore P, et al. The effect of halofuginone lactate on experimental *Cryptosporidium parvum* infections in calves. Vet Parasitol 1993;45:199–207.
[92] Villacorta I, Peeters JE, Vanopdenbosch E, et al. Efficacy of halofuginone lactate against *Cryptosporidium parvum* in calves. Antimicrob Agents Chemother 1991;35:283–7.
[93] Grinberg A, Markovics A, Galindez J, et al. Controlling the onset of natural cryptosporidiosis in calves with paromomycin sulphate. Vet Rec 2002;151:606–8.
[94] Viu M, Quilez J, Sanchez-Acedo C, et al. Field trial on the therapeutic efficacy of paromomycin on natural *Cryptosporidium parvum* infections in lambs. Vet Parasitol 2000;90:163–70.
[95] Fayer R, Ellis W. Paromomycin is effective as prophylaxis for cryptosporidiosis in dairy calves. J Parasitol 1993;79:771–4.
[96] Mancassola R, Richard A, Naciri M. Evaluation of decoquinate to treat experimental cryptosporidiosis in kids. Vet Parasitol 1997;69:31–7.
[97] Moore DA, Atwill ER, Kirk JH, et al. Prophylactic use of decoquinate for infections with *Cryptosporidium parvum* in experimentally challenged neonatal calves. J Am Vet Med Assoc 2003;223:839–45.
[98] de Graaf DC, Spano F, Petry F, et al. Speculation on whether a vaccine against cryptosporidiosis is a reality or fantasy. Int J Parasitol 1999;29:1289–306.
[99] Harp JA, Goff JP. Strategies for the control of Cryptosporidium parvum infection in calves. J Dairy Sci 1998;81:289–94.

ELSEVIER
SAUNDERS

Vet Clin Food Anim
22 (2006) 645–671

VETERINARY
CLINICS
Food Animal Practice

Neosporosis, Toxoplasmosis, and Sarcocystosis in Ruminants

J.P. Dubey, MVSc, PhD[a,*], David S. Lindsay, PhD[b]

[a]United States Department of Agriculture, Agricultural Research Service, Animal and Natural Resources Institute, Beltsville Agricultural Research Center, Building 1001, Beltsville, Maryland, 20705–2350, USA

[b]Department of Biomedical Sciences and Pathobiology, Virginia-Maryland Regional College of Veterinary Medicine, Virginia Tech, 1410 Prices Fork Road, Blacksburg, VA 24061–0342, USA

Neosporosis

Etiologic agent

Neosporosis is caused by the protozoan parasite, *Neospora caninum*. Until 1988, *N caninum* was confused with a closely related parasite, *Toxoplasma gondii* [1,2]. Since its first recognition as a clinical disease of dogs in Norway in 1984 [3], neosporosis has emerged as a serious disease of cattle and dogs worldwide [4–6]. Additionally, clinical neosporosis has been reported occasionally in other animals, and antibodies to *N caninum* have been found in the sera of many species of domestic and free-range land mammals as well as in marine mammals [7]. Until now, however, viable *N caninum* has been isolated only from dogs, cattle, white-tailed deer, water buffaloes, and sheep [7]. At present, there is no evidence that *N caninum* infects human beings.

N caninum is a coccidian parasite, and its oocysts have been found in feces of dogs and coyotes [8–13]. Thus, dogs are the intermediate and definitive host for *N caninum*. The life cycle is typified by three infectious stages: tachyzoites, tissue cysts, and oocysts (Fig. 1). Tachyzoites and tissue cysts are the stages found in the intermediate hosts, and they occur intracellularly [2]. Tachyzoites are approximately 6 μm × 2 μm. Tissue cysts are often round or oval in shape, up to 107 μm long, and are found primarily in

* Corresponding author.
E-mail address: jdubey@anri.barc.usda.gov (J.P. Dubey).

0749-0720/06/$ - see front matter. Published by Elsevier Inc.
doi:10.1016/j.cvfa.2006.08.001

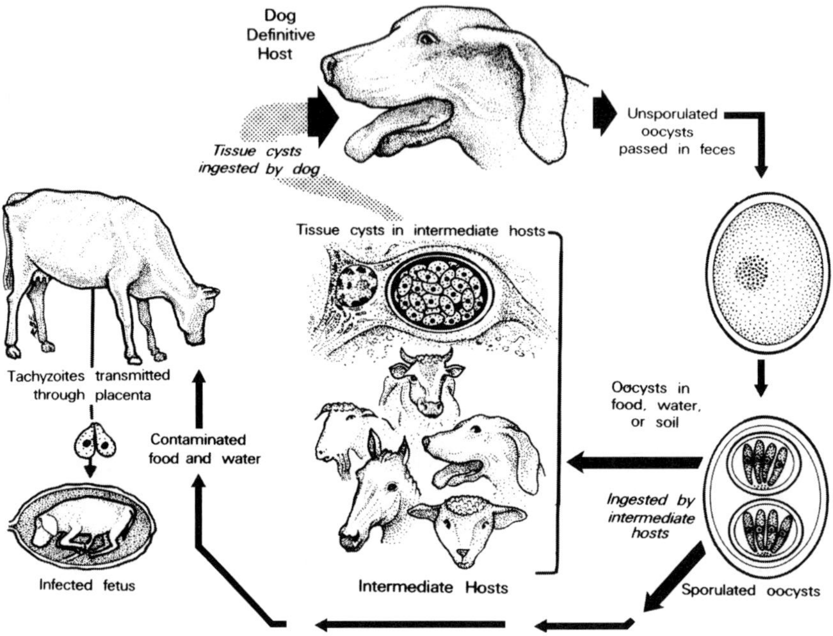

Fig. 1. Life cycle of *Neospora caninum*. (*From* Dubey JP. Review of *Neospora caninum* and neosporosis in animals. Korean J Parasitol 2003;41:1–16.)

the central nervous system (CNS). The tissue cyst wall is up to 4 μm thick, and the enclosed bradyzoites are 7 to 8 μm × 2 μm.

N caninum oocysts are excreted unsporulated in feces and measure approximately 12 μm in diameter, and sporulation occurs outside the host. At present, little is known regarding the frequency of shedding of oocysts, the survival of the oocysts in the environment, and whether other canids are also definitive hosts for *N caninum* [7]. The parasite can be transmitted transplacentally in several hosts, and the vertical route is the major mode of its transmission in cattle [14–16]. There is no cow-to-cow transmission of *N caninum*. Although most *N caninum* infections in cattle are transmitted transplacentally, postnatal rates have been variable depending on the region of the country, type of test used, and cutoff values used [7]. Although *N caninum* has been found in bovine semen [17], it is unlikely that *N caninum* is transmitted venereally or by embryo transfer from the donor cows. Actually, embryo transfer is even recommended as a method of control to prevent vertical transmission [18]. Nevertheless, it is prudent to test all recipients, and embryos should not be transferred to seropositive cows. Lactogenic transmission of *N caninum* is considered unlikely [19–21]. Carnivores can acquire infection by ingestion of infected tissues.

Neosporosis in cattle

Clinical signs

N caninum causes abortion in dairy and beef cattle [5,22–28]. Cows of any age may abort from 3 months of gestation to term. Most neosporosis-induced abortions occur at 5 to 6 months of gestation. Fetuses may die in utero, be resorbed, mummified, autolyzed, stillborn, born alive with clinical signs, or born clinically normal but chronically infected. Neosporosis-induced abortions occur year-round. Cows with *N caninum* antibodies (seropositive) are more likely to abort than seronegative cows, and this applies to dairy and beef cattle. Up to 95% of calves born congenitally infected from seropositive dams remain clinically normal, however. The age of the dam, lactation number, and history of abortion generally do not affect the rate of congenital infection, but there are reports indicating that vertical transmission is more efficient in younger than older cows in persistently infected cattle [16]. The infected replacement heifers may abort or transplacentally infect their offspring.

Clinical signs have only been reported in cattle younger than 2 month of age [5]. *N caninum*–infected calves may have neurologic signs, be underweight, be unable to rise, or be born without clinical signs of disease. Hind limbs, forelimbs, or both may be flexed or hyperextended. Neurologic examination may reveal ataxia, decreased patellar reflexes, and loss of conscious proprioception. Calves may have exophthalmia or an asymmetric appearance in the eyes. *N caninum* occasionally causes birth defects, including hydrocephalus and narrowing of the spinal cord [5].

Abortions may be epidemic or endemic [22–28]. Up to 33% of dairy cow fetuses have been reported to abort within a few months. Abortions are considered epidemic if more than 10% of cows at risk aborted within 6 to 8 weeks. A small proportion (<5%) of cows have been reported to have repeated abortion because of neosporosis [25]. Cows with *N caninum* antibodies (seropositive) are more likely to abort than seronegative cows. There is a rise in antibody titers 4 to 5 months before parturition. These observations strongly suggest reactivation of latent infection. Little is known of the mechanism of reactivation. It is likely that there is parasitemia during pregnancy, leading to fetal infection. *N caninum* has never been identified in histologic sections taken from adult cows, however, whereas viable *N caninum* has been isolated from the brain of only two cows [29,30]. Although it is reasonable to speculate that pregnancy-induced immune suppression or hormonal imbalance may reactivate latent tissue cysts of *N caninum*, such a mechanism has not been demonstrated for neosporosis. *N caninum* DNA has been found in blood of naturally infected cattle, indicating parasitemia [31]. *N caninum* is one of the most efficiently transplacentally transmitted organisms in cattle. In some herds, up to 90% of cattle are infected and most calves born congenitally infected with *N caninum* remain healthy.

Prevalence

N caninum infections have been reported from most parts of the world and seroprevalences for each host were tabulated recently [7]. Quantitative studies involving a large number of fetuses in many countries indicate that 12% to 42% of aborted fetuses from dairy cattle are infected with *N caninum* [7].

Serologic prevalence in cattle varies, depending on the country, region, type of serologic test used, and cutoff level used to determine the exposure. In some dairies, up to 87% of cows are seropositive [5,7].

In general, less is known about the causes of abortion in beef cattle than in dairy cattle because of the difficulty in finding small fetuses expelled in the first trimester. Therefore, there are no accurate assessments of *Neospora*-induced losses in beef cattle. Because clinical disease has not been reported in calves older than 2 months of age, there is no direct evidence of *N caninum*–associated morbidity in adult cattle.

Diagnosis

Examination of the serum from an aborting cow is only indicative of exposure to *N caninum*, and histologic examination of the fetus is necessary for a definitive diagnosis of neosporosis [32]. The brain, heart, liver, placenta, and body fluids or blood serum are the best specimens for diagnosis, and diagnostic rates are higher if multiple tissues are examined [33]. Although lesions of neosporosis are found in several organs, fetal brain is the most consistently affected organ [33]. Because most aborted fetuses are likely to be autolyzed, even semiliquid brain tissue should be fixed in 10% buffered neutral formalin for histologic examination of hematoxylin and eosin (H&E)–stained sections. Immunohistochemistry is necessary, because there are generally only a few *N caninum* present in autolyzed tissues and these are often not visible in H&E-stained sections. The most characteristic lesion of neosporosis is focal encephalitis characterized by necrosis and nonsuppurative inflammation [33]. Hepatitis is more common in epizootic than sporadic abortions [34]. Lesions are also present in the placenta but protozoa are difficult to find.

The efficiency of the diagnosis by polymerase chain reaction (PCR) is dependent on the laboratory, stage of the autolysis of the fetus, and sampling procedures [32,35,36]. Although immunohistochemical demonstration of *N caninum* in lesions is the best evidence for the etiology of abortion at the present time, it is quite insensitive. *N caninum* DNA can be detected by PCR in formalin-fixed paraffin-embedded bovine aborted brain tissue.

Several serologic tests can be used to detect *N caninum* antibodies, including various ELISAs, the indirect fluorescent antibody test (IFAT), and the *Neospora* agglutination test (NAT) [37–48]. There are several modifications of the ELISA to detect antibodies to *N caninum* in sera or milk using whole parasite, whole parasite lysate, purified proteins, recombinant proteins, and tachyzoite proteins absorbed on immune stimulating complexes (ISCOM) particles, and some of these tests were compared recently in a multicenter study in various laboratories in Europe [46]. Avidity ELISAs designed to distinguish recent and chronic infections in cattle seem to be promising to distinguish endemic and epidemic abortion [45]. In the avidity ELISA, sera are treated with urea to release low-avidity (low-affinity) antibodies, and differences in values obtained before and after treatment with urea are used to evaluate recency of infection. In recently acquired infection, avidity values are low [45]. Another modification of the ELISA is the antigen-capture ELISA (cELISA). This test detects (captures) a 65-kd antigen in sera of infected cattle using a specific monoclonal antibody, and this test is commercially available [47,48]. Immunoblots are useful in detecting *N caninum*–specific antibodies [32].

Finding *N caninum* antibody in serum from the fetus can establish *N caninum* infection, but a negative result is not informative, because antibody synthesis in the fetus is dependent on the stage of gestation, level of exposure, and time between infection and abortion. Immunoblotting using *N caninum*–specific antigen improves diagnosis. Although blood serum or any body fluid from the fetus may be used for serologic diagnosis, peritoneal fluid is better than other body fluids. In calves, presuckling serum can be submitted for diagnosis of congenital infection.

The definitive antibody level that should be considered diagnostic for neosporosis has not been established for bovine species because of the uncertainty of serologic diagnosis in chronically infected animals and the availability of sera from noninfected cattle. In serologic assays, titer and absorbance values are dependent on antigen composition, secondary antibodies, and other reagents [32]. In addition, cutoff levels can be arbitrarily selected to provide sensitivity and specificity requested for a particular application. The age and class of an animal may also affect selection of a cutoff level. Although *N caninum* is closely related to *T gondii*, *Sarcocystis* species, and other apicomplexans, cross-reactivity has not been a major issue. In general, antibody titers are higher in cattle that have aborted because of neosporosis than in those with a normal pregnancy; however, titers in individual cows cannot determine the etiology of abortions.

Control

N caninum is efficiently transmitted vertically in cattle, perhaps for several generations. Therefore, culling is one way at present to prevent this transmission from cow to heifer [49,50]. Culling is not practical if the prevalence of *N caninum* in a herd is extremely high, however. Before making a decision to cull, it is advisable to estimate the prevalence of *N caninum* in the herd. Bulk milk testing can provide the preliminary information about the presence of *N caninum* infection. If a bulk milk test is positive, antibody prevalence in dam-heifer samples and cattle of different ages can provide insight into the transmission of *N caninum* in a given herd. In herds with high transplacental transmission, the prevalence of *N caninum* in cattle of different ages is about the same and there is a high correlation between infection in dams and daughters. To reduce vertical transmission of *N caninum*, culling of seropositive dams and/or heifer calves from seropositive cows and embryo transfer from seropositive cows to seronegative cows are two of the methods that can be adapted. Drugs that kill encysted *N caninum* in bovine tissues are unknown.

To prevent horizontal (from outside sources) transmission, it is important to prevent exposure of the cows to feed and water contaminated with oocysts [51–53]. Dogs and other canids should not be allowed in cattle barns or pasture, although this is not always easy to achieve. How dogs become infected with *N caninum* is not known. Consumption of aborted bovine fetuses does not seem to be an important source of *N caninum* infection in dogs. The consumption of placental membranes may be a source of *N caninum* infection in dogs because the parasite has been found in naturally infected placentas and dogs fed placentas shed *N caninum* oocysts [21]. Little is known at present regarding the frequency of shedding of *N caninum* oocysts by canids in nature, the resistance of the oocysts, and whether dogs shed oocysts more than once. Until more definitive hosts of *N caninum* are found, dogs and coyotes should not be allowed to eat aborted fetuses, fetal membranes, or dead calves. Other factors, such as farm location, can also be a risk [53]. Drugs that prevent transmission of the parasite from the dam to the fetus are unknown, but research is continuing in this area.

There is evidence that cattle can develop protective immunity to subsequent neosporosis abortion [54–57]. This protective immunity seems to be more effective in cows that are subsequently infected with an exogenous source (oocysts) than in cows in which there is a recrudescence of persistent infection [56]. Therefore, to elicit protective immunity against abortion in cows that already harbor a latent infection is a problem.

Currently, there is a killed-parasite commercial *N caninum* vaccine (Neo Guard), but there are no convincing data about the efficiency of this vaccine to prevent *N caninum*–associated abortion in cattle [58,59].

Neosporosis in other animals

Neosporosis is a primary disease of dogs. In addition to dogs and cattle, sporadic cases of clinical neosporosis have been reported in other animals, including adult horses, a 16-day-old rhinoceros (*Ceratotherium simum*), a juvenile raccoon (*Procyon lotor*), a 2-month-old black-tailed deer (*Odocoileus hemionus columbianus*), neonatal alpacas (*Vicugna pacos*) and llamas (*Lama glama*), goats, sheep, Eld's deer (*Cervus eldi siamensis*), fallow deer (*Dama dama*), and an antelope (*Tragelaphus imberbis*) [7]. A new species, *Neospora hughesi*, has been described in horses [60]. It is uncertain whether *N caninum* infects horses.

Toxoplasmosis

Etiologic agent

Toxoplasmosis is caused by the infection with the protozoan *T gondii* [61]. It is among the most common parasites of animals, and *T gondii* is the only known species. Felids are the definitive hosts, and warm-blooded animals are intermediate hosts [62]. There are three infectious stages of *T gondii* for all hosts: tachyzoites (individually and in groups), bradyzoites (in tissue cysts), and sporozoites (in oocysts) (Fig. 2).

The tachyzoite is often crescent shaped and 2 μm × 6 μm in size. It enters the host cell by active penetration of the cell membrane and becomes surrounded by a parasitophorous vacuole that protects it from host defense mechanisms. The tachyzoite multiplies asexually by repeated binary divisions until the host cell ruptures. After an unknown numbers of divisions, *T gondii* tachyzoites give rise to another stage called a tissue cyst. Tissue cysts grow and remain intracellular. They vary in size from 5 to 70 μm and contain a few to several hundred bradyzoites [63]. Although tissue cysts may develop in visceral organs, including the lungs, liver, and kidneys, they are more prevalent

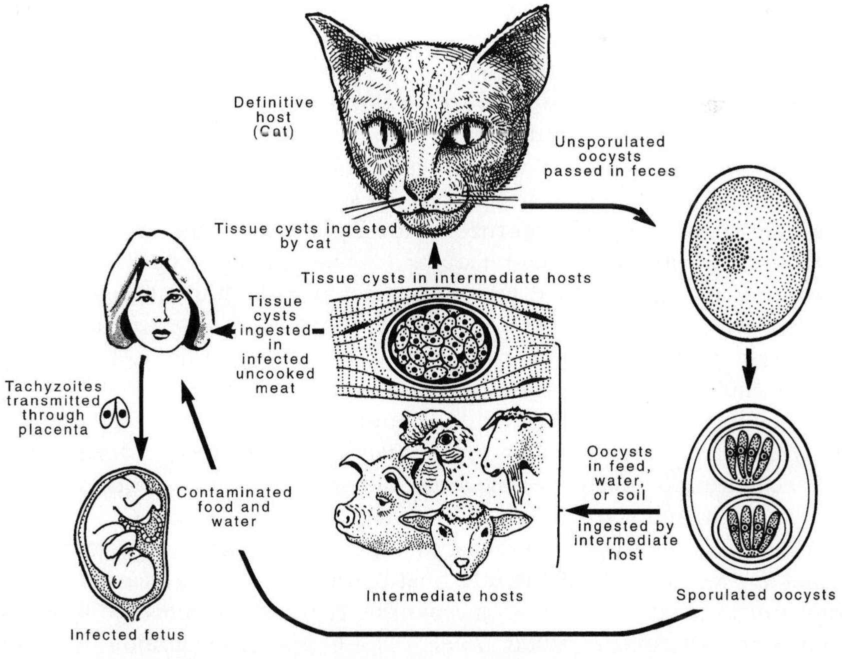

Fig. 2. Life cycle of *Toxoplasma gondii*. (*From* Dubey JP. Toxoplasmosis-a waterborne zoonosis. Vet Parasitol 2004;126:57–72.)

in muscular and neural tissues, including the brain, eye, and skeletal and cardiac muscle. Intact tissue cysts are probably harmless and can persist for the life of the host [63]. The tissue cyst wall is elastic and thin (<0.5 μm), and it may enclose hundreds of crescent-shaped slender bradyzoites, each measuring 7 μm × 1.5 μm. Bradyzoites differ only slightly from tachyzoites in having a nucleus situated toward the posterior end, whereas the nucleus in tachyzoites is more central. Additionally, bradyzoites are more slender than tachyzoites and less susceptible to destruction by proteolytic enzymes.

On ingestion by cats, the wall of the tissue cyst is digested by the proteolytic enzymes in the stomach and small intestine and bradyzoites are released. Some penetrate the lamina propria of the intestine and multiple as tachyzoites. Within a few hours, *T gondii* may disseminate to extraintestinal tissues. Other bradyzoites penetrate epithelial cells of the small intestine and initiate development of numerous generations of asexual (types A–E) schizonts [64,65]. The organisms (merozoites) released from schizonts form male and female gametes. After the female gamete is fertilized by the male gamete, oocyst wall formation begins around the fertilized gamete. When oocysts are mature, they are discharged into the intestinal lumen by the rupture of intestinal epithelial cells. *T gondii* persists in the intestinal and extraintestinal tissue of cats for at least several months, and possibly for the life of the cat.

Oocysts of *T gondii* are formed only in cats, including domestic and wild felids. Cats shed oocysts after ingesting tachyzoites, bradyzoites, or sporozoites [62,64,66–70]. Less than 50% of cats shed oocysts after ingesting tachyzoites or oocysts, however, whereas nearly all shed oocysts after ingesting tissue cysts [66,68–70].

Oocysts in freshly passed feces are unsporulated (noninfective), subspherical to spherical in shape, and 10 μm × 12 μm in diameter. Sporulation occurs outside the cat and within 1 to 5 days depending on aeration and temperature. Sporulated oocysts contain two ellipsoidal sporocysts. Each sporocyst contains four sporozoites. The sporozoites are 2 μm × 6 to 8 μm in size.

Hosts, including felids, can acquire *T gondii* by ingesting tissues of infected animals or food or drink contaminated with sporulated oocysts or by transplacental transmission. After ingestion, bradyzoites released from tissue cysts or sporozoites from oocysts penetrate intestinal tissues, transform to tachyzoites, multiply locally, and are disseminated in the body via blood or lymph. After a few multiplication cycles, tachyzoites give rise to bradyzoites in a variety of tissues. *Toxoplasma gondii* infection during pregnancy can lead to infection of the fetus. Congenital toxoplasmosis in human beings, sheep, and goats can kill the fetus.

After ingestion of sporulated oocysts, sporozoites excyst, penetrate enterocytes and goblet cells of the intestinal epithelium, and are carried to the lamina propria via an unknown mechanism. Some sporozoites can be found circulating in peripheral blood as early as 4 hours after ingestion. Most remain in the lamina propria, however, where they multiply in a variety of cells, including vascular endothelium, fibroblasts, mononuclear cells, and segmented leukocytes, but not in erythrocytes. Edema, necrosis of the lamina propria, and sloughing of the intestinal mucosa can produce severe enteritis. Infection can eventually spread to all other organs.

Host-parasite relation

T gondii can multiply in most mammalian cells. How it is destroyed by immune cells is not completely known. All extracellular forms of the parasite are directly affected by antibodies, but intracellular forms are not. Cellular factors, including lymphocytes and lymphokines, are thought to be more important than humoral factors in the immune-mediated destruction of *T gondii.*

Immunity does not eliminate an established infection. *T gondii* tissue cysts persist several years after acute infection. The ultimate fate of tissue cysts is not fully known. Some may rupture during the life of the host, and the released bradyzoites may be destroyed by the host's immune responses. In immunosuppressed individuals, however, infection can be reactivated by dissemination of bradyzoites and conversion to tachyzoites.

The pathogenicity of *T gondii* is determined by many factors, including the susceptibility of the host species, virulence of the parasitic strain, and stage. Oocyst-induced infections are the most clinically severe in intermediate hosts, and this is not dose dependent [61]. *T gondii* isolates differ remarkably in their virulence to outbred mice, but virulence of *T gondii* in mice should not be equated with virulence in human beings or domestic animals. *T gondii* has also adapted to an oocyst-oral cycle in herbivores (intermediate hosts) and to a tissue cyst–oral cycle in carnivores, especially in the cat. *T gondii* oocysts are less infective and less pathogenic for the cat than for mice [67,70]. For example, 1 live oocyst is orally infective to mice and pigs [71], whereas 100 or more oocysts may be required to establish infection in a cat [70]. The reverse may be true for bradyzoites. By mouth, bradyzoites are less infective to mice than cats [72]. Cats can shed millions of oocysts after ingesting as few as 1 bradyzoite, whereas 100 bradyzoites may not be infective to mice by the oral route [70,72]. Although *T gondii* can be transmitted orally by ingesting tissue cysts, epidemiologic evidence indicates that cats are essential in perpetuation of the life cycle, because *T gondii* infection is rare or absent in areas devoid of cats [73–75].

Epidemiology

Domestic cats are probably the major source of contamination, because they are common and produce large numbers of *T gondii* oocysts [64,72]. Sporulated oocysts survive for long periods under moderate environmental conditions. For example, they can survive in moist soil for months to years [61]. Oocysts in soil can be spread mechanically by flies, cockroaches, dung beetles, and earthworms. Oocysts are known to survive on fruits and vegetables for long periods [76]. Humans may acquire toxoplasmosis by petting dogs that have rolled over in infected cat feces [77–79].

Although only a few cats may be shedding *T gondii* oocysts at any given time, the enormous numbers produced and their resistance to destruction ensure widespread contamination [80]. Latently infected cats can shed oocysts after challenge infection. Congenitally infected kittens can also excrete oocysts. Infection rates in cats are largely determined by the rate of infection in the local avian and rodent populations that serve as a food source. For epidemiologic surveys, seroprevalence data for cats are more useful than results of fecal examination, because cats with antibodies have probably already shed oocysts and are an indicator of environmental contamination [64].

Infection in human beings is probably most often the result of ingestion of tissue cysts contained in raw or undercooked meat, because *T gondii* is common in many animals used for food, including sheep, pigs, and rabbits. Viable *T gondii* has not been isolated from beef, and the role of cattle in the transmission of infection to human beings is at best uncertain [81]. Although the prevalence of *T gondii* in pigs raised under good management practices has decreased drastically [81], infection rates can be high in pigs raised outdoors and in unhygienic conditions [82]. Tissue cysts can survive in food animals for years [61]. Virtually all edible portions of carcasses can be infected with viable *T gondii.*

Cultural habits may also affect the acquisition of *T gondii* infection. The high incidence of *T gondii* infection in human beings in France seems to be related, in part, to the French habit of eating some meat raw. In contrast, the high prevalence of the infection in Central America and South America is in probably attributable to high levels of contamination of the environment by oocysts [83]. Outbreaks of acute toxoplasmosis have been reported in human beings by drinking water contaminated with oocysts [84,85]. It should be noted, however, that the relative frequency of acquisition of toxoplasmosis from eating raw meat and that attributable to ingestion of food contaminated by oocysts from cat feces in the general population are unknown. At present, there are no tests to distinguish oocyst- versus meat-acquired *T gondii* infection.

In addition to infection as a result of ingestion of oocysts and by eating infected raw meat, transmission of toxoplasmosis can be by semen transfusion, by ingestion of milk or saliva, and by eating eggs. The stages most likely to be involved in these transmissions are tachyzoites, which are not environmentally resistant and are killed by water. The probability of transmission of *T gondii* by these means is rare, however. There is little if any danger of *T gondii* infection by drinking cow's milk, which, in any case, is generally pasteurized or even boiled, but infection has followed drinking unboiled goat's milk. Raw hens' eggs, although an important source of *Salmonella* infection, are extremely unlikely to harbor *T gondii.* Transmission by sexual activity, including kissing, is probably rare and epidemiologically unimportant.

Transmission can also occur through blood transfusions and organ transplants, with transplantation being the more important; this is a recent development. In people undergoing transplantation, toxoplasmosis may arise from implantation of an organ or bone marrow from an infected donor into a nonimmune immunocompromised recipient or from induction of disease in an immunocompromised latently infected recipient. The tissue cysts in the transplanted tissue or in the latently infected person are probably the source of the infection. In both cases, the cytotoxic and immunosuppressive therapy given to the recipient is the cause of the induction of the active infection and the disease.

Clinical toxoplasmosis

T gondii is capable of causing severe disease in animals other than human beings [61] and is responsible for great losses to the livestock industry. In sheep and goats, it may cause embryonic death and resorption, fetal death and mummification, abortion, stillbirth, and neonatal death. Disease is more severe in goats than in sheep. Outbreaks of toxoplasmosis in pigs have been reported from several countries, especially Japan, and mortality is more common in young pigs than in adult pigs. Pneumonia, myocarditis, encephalitis, and placental necrosis occur in infected pigs. Cattle and horses are more resistant to clinical toxoplasmosis than are other species of livestock; there is no confirmed report of clinical toxoplasmosis in cattle, horses, and water buffaloes. In cats and dogs, the disease is most severe in young animals. Common clinical manifestations of canine toxoplasmosis are respiratory distress, ataxia, and diarrhea. In most infected dogs, pneumonia is caused by a combination of *T gondii* and distemper virus, because the virus is immunosuppressive. Respiratory distress is a common clinical sign in cats with toxoplasmosis. Although cats of any age can die of toxoplasmosis, kittens and those with depressed immunity are the most likely victims [86,87].

Sporadic and widespread outbreaks of toxoplasmosis occur in rabbits, mink, birds, and other domesticated and wild animals [61,88–91]. Toxoplasmosis is severe in many species of Australian marsupials and in marsupials, New World monkeys, Pallas cats, and canaries.

Free-ranging marine mammals have died of acute toxoplasmosis [92]. Numerous reports exist of *T gondii* infections in marine mammals, including sea otters, dolphins, seals, and whales [92], and toxoplasmosis has been considered a cause of death in sea otters [93–95]; yet, how marine mammals become infected is unknown. Cole and colleagues [93] postulated, based on clinical evidence in sea otters, and Miller and coworkers [95] presented evidence that coastal fresh water surface runoff presented a risk of infection to sea otters; thus, it is possible that *T gondii* oocysts could be washed into the sea via runoff contaminated by cat excrement.*T gondii* infection is widespread in human beings, and the prevalence varies with geography and increase in age. In the United States and the United Kingdom, it is estimated that 16% to 40% of people become infected, whereas in Central American and South America and continental Europe, infection estimates reach 50% to 80% [61,88,96]. Infections in healthy adults are usually asymptomatic; however, severe disease can occur in immunocompromised individuals and newborns.

Congenital infection may occur after maternal infection during pregnancy. The severity of the disease may depend on the stage of pregnancy at the time of infection. A wide spectrum of clinical disease occurs in congenitally infected children [97,98]. Mild disease may consist of slightly diminished vision only, whereas severely diseased children may have the full tetrad of signs, including retinochoroiditis, hydrocephalus, convulsions, and intracerebral calcification. Of these, hydrocephalus is the least common but most dramatic lesion of toxoplasmosis. This condition is unique to congenitally acquired toxoplasmosis in human beings and has not been reported in other animals.

Postnatally acquired infection may be localized or generalized. Oocyst-transmitted infections may be more severe than tissue cyst–induced infections [84,85]. Lymphadenitis is the most frequently observed clinical form of toxoplasmosis in human beings [61,84]. Although any nodes may be involved, the most frequently involved are the deep cervical nodes. When infected, they are tender and discrete but not painful, and the infections resolve spontaneously in weeks or months. Lymphadenopathy may be associated with fever, malaise, fatigue, muscle pain, and sore throat and headache. Although the condition may be benign, its diagnosis is vital in pregnant women because of the risk to the fetus. Many patients with AIDS and those given immunosuppressive treatments die of acute toxoplasmosis, often involving brain [99].

Diagnosis

Diagnosis is made by biologic, serologic, or histologic methods or by some combination of these. Clinical signs are nonspecific and insufficiently characteristic for a definite diagnosis, because toxoplasmosis mimics several other infectious diseases.

Numerous serologic procedures are available for the detection of humoral antibodies, including the Sabin-Feldman dye test, indirect hemagglutination assays, IFATs, direct agglutination tests, latex agglutination tests, ELISAs, and the immunoabsorbent agglutination assay test (ISAAGA) [61,98]. The IFAT, ISAAGA, and ELISAs have been modified to detect IgM antibodies, which appear sooner after infection than IgG antibodies and disappear faster than IgG antibodies after recovery.

The finding of antibodies to *T gondii* in one serum sample merely establishes that the host has been infected at some time in the past; thus, it is best to collect two samples from the same individual, the second 2 to 4 weeks after the first. A 4- to 16-fold increase in antibody titers in the second sample indicates an acute infection. A high antibody titer sometimes persists for months after infection. A rise in antibody titers may not be associated with clinical symptoms, because, as indicated earlier, most infections in human beings are asymptomatic and the fact that titers persist after clinical recovery complicates the interpretation of the results of serologic tests. *T gondii* can be isolated from patients by inoculation into laboratory animals and tissue cultures of secretions, excretions, body fluids, tissues taken by biopsy, and tissues with macroscopic lesions taken after death. Using such specimens, it is possible not only to attempt isolation of *T gondii* but to search for *T gondii* microscopically or for toxoplasmic DNA using the PCR for processing. It is advisable not to rely entirely on this test for making vital decisions involving the fetus.

As just noted, diagnosis can be made by finding *T gondii* in host tissue removed by biopsy or at necropsy. A rapid diagnosis may be made by microscopic examination of impression smears of lesions. After drying for 10 to 30 minutes, the smears are fixed in methyl alcohol and stained with a Romanowsky stain, with a Giemsa stain being satisfactory. Well-preserved *T gondii* are crescent shaped. In sections, the tachyzoites usually appear round to oval. Electron microscopy can aid in diagnosis. *T gondii* tachyzoites are always located in vacuoles; they have few (usually four) rhoptries and often have a honeycomb structure. Tissue cysts are usually spherical and lack septa, and the cyst wall stains with silver stains. The bradyzoites are strongly periodic acid–Schiff (PAS)-positive [61]. The immunohistochemical staining of parasites with fluorescent or other types of labeled *T gondii* antiserum can aid in diagnosis.

Chemotherapy

Sulfadiazine and pyrimethamine are widely used for therapy of toxoplasmosis [61,100]. These drugs act synergistically by blocking the metabolic pathway involving *p*-aminobenzoic acid and the folic-folinic acid cycle, respectively. The drugs are usually well tolerated; sometimes, thrombocytopenia or leukopenia may develop, but these effects can be overcome by administering folinic acid and yeast without interfering with treatment, because the vertebrate host can transport presynthesized folinic acid into its cells, whereas *T gondii* cannot. Although these drugs have a beneficial action when given in the acute stage of the disease when there is active multiplication of the parasite, they do not usually eradicate infection. These drugs seem to have little effect on subclinical infections, but the growth of tissue cysts in mice has been restrained with sulfonamides. Sulfa compounds are excreted within a few hours of administration; thus, treatment has to be administered in daily divided doses. Doses vary with age and the species of the host [100,101]. Spiramycin, clindamycin, atovaquone, azithromycin, roxithromycin, clarithromycin, dapsone, and several other less commonly used drugs are available for treatment of toxoplasmosis. Clindamycin is absorbed quickly and diffuses well into the CNS; therefore, it has been used as an alternative to sulfadiazine [101].

Prevention and control

To prevent infection of human beings by *T gondii*, people handling meat should wash their hands thoroughly with soap and water before going to other tasks [61,102]. All cutting boards, sink tops, knives, and other materials contacting uncooked meat should also be washed with soap and water. Washing is effective because the stages of *T gondii* in meat are killed by contact with soap and water [61]. *T gondii* in meat is killed by exposure to extreme cold or heat. Tissue cysts in meat are killed by heating to an internal temperature of 67°C [103] or by cooling to −13°C [104]. *T gondii* in tissue cysts or oocysts is killed by exposure to 0.5 kilorads of γ-irradiation [105,106]. Meat of any animal should be cooked to a minimum of 67°C before consumption, and tasting meat while cooking or while seasoning should be avoided. High-pressure treatment can kill tissue cysts in meat and oocysts on fruits and vegetables [107,108]. Salt additives to tenderize the meat can reduce inactivate tissue cysts in meat [81,109].

Pregnant women should avoid contact with cats, cat litter, soil, and raw meat. Pet cats should be fed only dry, canned, or cooked food, and the cat litter box should be emptied daily. Gloves should be worn while gardening, and vegetables should be washed thoroughly before eating because they may have been contaminated with cat feces. People should avoid drinking unfiltered water from lakes, ponds, and rivers. Access to water reservoirs by cats should be prevented.

Vaccination

There is no commercial vaccine to prevent *T gondii* infection in cats and human beings. One vaccine that contains a strain (S48) of tachyzoites that does not persist in the tissues of sheep is available in Europe and New Zealand, where it is used to reduce fetal losses attributable to toxoplasmosis [110]. Ewes vaccinated with the S48 strain vaccine retain immunity for at least 18 months [110].

Sarcocystosis

Etiologic agent

Unlike *Neospora* and *Toxoplasma*, the genus *Sarcocystis* has more than 100 species that infect mammals, birds, marsupials, and poikilothermic animals. *Sarcocystis* has an obligatory prey-predator (two-host) life cycle (Fig. 3). Asexual stages develop only in the intermediate host, which, in nature, is often a prey animal, and sexual stages develop only in the definitive host, which is carnivorous. There are different intermediate and definitive hosts for each species of *Sarcocystis*; for example, there are three named species of *Sarcocystis* in cattle: *Sarcocystis cruzi*, *Sarcocystis hirsuta*, and *Sarcocystis hominis* [111], with the definitive hosts for these species being Canidae,

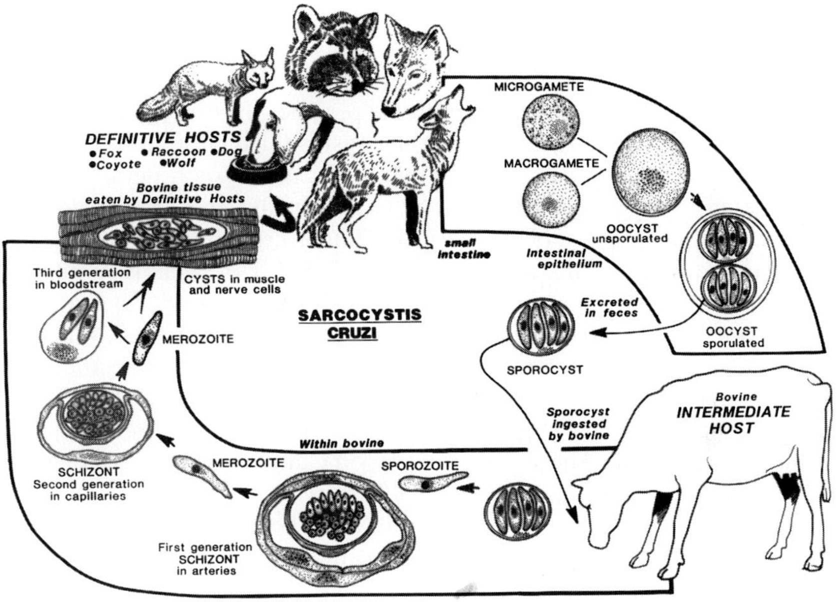

Fig. 3. Life cycle of *Sarcocystis cruzi*. (*From* Dubey JP, Fayer R. Bovine sarcocystosis. Comp Contin Edu Pract Vet 1986;8:130–42.)

Felidae, and primates, respectively. Species of *Sarcocystis* are generally more specific for their intermediate hosts than for their definitive hosts; for *S cruzi*, for example, ox and bison are the only intermediate hosts, whereas dogs, wolves, coyotes, raccoons, jackals, and foxes can act as definitive hosts. In the following description of life cycle and structure, *S cruzi* serves as the example because its complete life cycle is known.

The intermediate host becomes infected by ingesting sporocysts in food or water. Sporozoites excyst from sporocysts in the small intestine, and first-generation schizonts are formed in endothelial cells of arteries 7 to 15 days after inoculation. Second-generation schizonts occur 19 to 46 days after inoculation, predominantly in capillaries virtually throughout the body. Merozoites are found in mononuclear blood cells 24 to 46 days after inoculation.

The schizonts divide by endopolygeny, wherein the nucleus becomes lobulated and divides into several nuclei. Merozoites form at the periphery of the schizont. First- and second-generation schizonts are located within the host cytoplasm and are not surrounded by a parasitophorous vacuole. *Sarcocystis* merozoites have the same organelles as do other coccidians, but there are no rhoptries. Rhoptries, however, are present in *Sarcocystis* bradyzoites [111].

Merozoites liberated from the terminal vascular generation of the developing parasite initiate sarcocyst formation. These merozoites penetrate appropriate host cells. The intracellular merozoite, which is surrounded by a parasitophorous vacuole (PV), becomes round to ovoid (metrocyte) and undergoes repeated division, producing many metrocytes that eventually produce banana-shaped zoites called bradyzoites (also called cystozoites). Some mature sarcocysts may contain some peripherally arranged metrocytes in addition to zoites. Eventually, the sarcocyst is filled with bradyzoites, the stage infective for the predator definitive host. Sarcocysts generally become infectious approximately 75 days after infection, but there is considerable variation among species of *Sarcocystis*. Immature sarcocysts containing only metrocytes and schizonts are not infectious for the definitive host.

The definitive host becomes infected by ingesting tissues containing mature sarcocysts. Bradyzoites liberated from the sarcocyst by digestion in the stomach and intestine penetrate the mucosa of the small intestine and transform into male (micro) and female (macro) gamonts. After fertilization of a macrogamete by a microgamete, a wall develops around the zygote and an oocyst is formed. The entire process of gametogony and fertilization can be completed within 24 hours.

Oocysts of *Sarcocystis* species sporulate in the lamina propria. Sporulated oocysts are thin walled (<1 μm). The thin oocyst wall often ruptures, releasing the sporocysts into the intestinal lumen, from which they are passed in the feces. The prepatent and patent periods vary, but for most *Sarcocystis* species, oocysts are first shed in feces 7 to 14 days after ingesting sarcocysts.

The number of generations of schizogony and the type of host cell in which schizogony may occur vary with each species of *Sarcocystis*, but trends are apparent. For example, all species of *Sarcocystis* of large domestic animals (sheep, goats, cattle, and pigs) form first- and second-generation schizonts in the vascular endothelium, whereas only a single precystic generation of schizogony has been found in *Sarcocystis* species of small mammals (mice and deer mice), and this is generally in hepatocytes [111].

Sarcocysts, which are always located within a PV in the host cell cytoplasm, consist of a cyst wall that surrounds the metrocyte or the bradyzoites. The structure and thickness of the cyst wall differ among species of *Sarcocystis* and within each species as the sarcocyst matures [111]. Histologically, the sarcocyst wall may be smooth, striated, or hirsute, or it may possess complex branched protrusions. These protrusions are of taxonomic importance. Internally, groups of zoites may be segregated into compartments by septa that originate from the sarcocyst wall, or they may not be compartmentalized.

Not all species of *Sarcocystis* cause disease in their host species [111]. Generally, species using canids as definitive hosts are more pathogenic than those using felids. For example, of the three species in cattle, *S cruzi*, for which the dog is the definitive host, is the most pathogenic, whereas *S hirsuta* and *S hominis*, which undergo sexual development in cats and primates, respectively, are only mildly pathogenic (Table 1). Pathogenicity is manifested in the intermediate host. *Sarcocystis* generally does not cause illness in definitive hosts.

S neurona is an unusual species of the genus that does not follow the life cycle pattern of *S cruzi* outlined previously [112]. It is also one of the most pathogenic species of the genus. *S neurona* is the most frequent cause of a fatal disease in horses called equine protozoal encephalomyelitis (EPM) in North America and South America [112]. Horses are considered an aberrant host, because only schizonts are found in their tissues. Unlike *S cruzi*, *S neurona* schizonts occur in neural cells rather than in the vascular endothelium, and schizonts may persist in the CNS for months. Its sarcocysts occur in domestic cats, striped skunks, raccoons, sea otters, and armadillos. Opossums (*Didelphis virginianus* and *Didelphis abbreventis*) are its definitive hosts. Only the sexual cycle occurs in the definitive host, and it is confined to the small intestine. Encephalomyelitis associated with *S neurona* has been reported in horses, ponies, zebras, skunks, raccoons, cats, dogs, lynx, mink and marine mammals [112,113].

S canis is another unusual species of the genus with an unknown life cycle [113]. Its sarcocysts, sexual phase, and definitive hosts are unknown. The schizont is the only stage that is known. *S canis* has been found associated with fatal hepatitis in sea lions, dogs, black bears, grizzly bears, a horse, and a dolphin. Congenital infection has been documented in dogs.

Clinical sarcocystosis in animals

Sarcocystis is generally nonpathogenic for the definitive host, and some species of *Sarcocystis* are also nonpathogenic for intermediate hosts (see Table 1). Generally, species transmitted by canids are pathogenic, whereas those transmitted by felids are nonpathogenic. *S cruzi, Sarcocystis capracanis*, and *Sarcocystis tenella* are the most pathogenic species for cattle, goats, and sheep, respectively. Clinical signs are generally seen during the second schizogonic cycle in blood vessels (acute phase). Three to 4 weeks after infection with a large dose of sporocysts (50,000 or more), fever, anorexia, anemia, emaciation, and hair loss (particularly on the rump and tail in cattle) develop, and some animals die. Pregnant animals may abort, and growth is slowed or arrested. Animals recover as sarcocysts begin to mature.

Dramatic gross lesions are seen in animals that die during the acute phase. Edema, hemorrhage, and atrophy of fat are commonly seen. The hemorrhages are most evident on the serosa of viscera, in cardiac and skeletal muscle, and in the sclera of the eyes. Hemorrhages vary from petechiae to ecchymoses several centimeters in diameter. Microscopic lesions may be seen in many organs and consist of necrosis, edema, and infiltrations of mononuclear cells. During the chronic phase, lesions are restricted to muscles and consist of nonsuppurative myositis and degeneration of sarcocysts.

Clinical sarcocystosis in human beings

Human beings serve as the definitive host for *S hominis* and *Sarcocystis suihominis* and also serve as accidental intermediate hosts for several

Table 1
Sarcocystis species in livestock

Intermediate host	*Sarcocystis* species	Reference	Sarcocysts: Maximum length (mm)	Sarcocysts: Wall (mm)	Pathogenicity[a]	Definitive hosts
Cattle (*Bos taurus*)	*S cruzi*	Hasselmann, 1926; Wenyon, 1926	<1	7	++	Dog, coyote, red fox, raccoon, wolf
	S hirsuta	Moulé, 1888	7	10	+/−	Cat
	S hominis	Railliet and Lucet, 1891; Dubey, 1976	7	10	+/−	Man, other primates
Sheep (*Ovis aries*)	*S tenella*	Railliet, 1886; Moulé, 1886	0.7	14	++	Dog, coyote, red fox
	S arieticanis	Heydorn, 1985	0.9	7	+	Dog
	S gigantea	Railliet, 1886; Ashford, 1977	10	21	−	Cat
	S medusiformis	Collins et al, 1979	8	20	−	Cat
Goat (*Capra hircus*)	*S capracanis*	Fisher, 1979	1	14	++	Dog, coyote, red fox
	S hircicanis	Heydorn and Unterhozner, 1983	2.5	7	++	Dog
	S moule	Nevu-Nemaire, 1912	7.5	7	?	Cat
Pigs (*Sus scrofa*)	*S miescheriana*	Künn, 1865; Labbé, 1899	1.5	10 (?)	+	Dog, raccoon, wolf, red fox, jackal
	S porcifelis	Dubey, 1976	?	?	?	Cat
	S suihominis	Tadros and Laarman, 1976; Heydorn, 1977	1.5	10	+	Humans, primates

Horses (*Equus caballus*)	*S fayeri*	Dubey et al, 1977	1.0	11	+/−	Dog
	S equicanis	Rommel and Geisel, 1975	0.35	?	?	Dog
	S bertrami	Doflein, 1901	12	?	?	Dog
Water buffalo (*Bubalus bubalis*)	*S levinei*	Dissanike and Kan, 1978; Huong et al, 1997	1.1	7 (?)	+	Dog
	S fusiformis	Railliet, 1897; Bernard and Bauche, 1912	3	21	−	Cat
	S dubeyi	Huong and Uggla, 1999	<1 (?)	9	?	?
	S buffalonis	Huong et al, 1997	8	7.7	?	Cat
Camel (*Camelus spp*)	*S cameli*	Mason, 1910	0.38	?	?	Dog
	S sp	Mason, 1910	?	?	?	?
Chickens (*Gallus gallus*)	*S horvathi*	Ratz, 1908	0.98	?	?	?
	S sp	Wenzel, et al, 1982	?	?	?	Dog, cat
	S rileyi	Stiles, 1893; Minchin, 1903	12	23	?	Skunk

Abbreviations: + +, very pathogenic; +, pathogenic; mildly pathogenic; −, nonpathogenic; +/−, questionable pathogenicity; ?, unknown or unclassified.

[a] Modified from references [111,114], where a complete bibliography can be found.

unidentified species of *Sarcocystis* [111,114]. Symptoms vary with the species of *Sarcocystis* causing the infection and organ parasitized. Intestinal sarcocystosis is acquired by ingesting uncooked beef containing sarcocysts of *S hominis* or pork containing *S suihominis*. Symptoms include nausea, stomachache, and abdominal pain. Human volunteers developed hypersensitivity-like symptoms, including nausea, vomiting, stomachache, diarrhea, and dyspnea, within 24 hours of ingestion of uncooked pork from naturally or experimentally infected pigs. Sporocysts were shed 11 to 13 days after ingesting the infected pork or beef [114–121] Sarcocysts have been found in striated muscles of human beings, mostly as incidental findings [122]. Recently, 7 of 15 US military men developed acute illness after an army exercise in rural Malaysia [123]. The illness was characterized by fever, myalgias, bronchospasm, fleeting pruritic rashes, transient lymphadenopathy, and subcutaneous nodules associated with eosinophilia, an elevated erythrocyte sedimentation rate, and elevated levels of muscle creatinine kinase. Sarcocysts of an unidentified *Sarcocystis* species were found in skeletal muscle biopsies of the index case [123].

Eosinophilic myositis

Eosinophilic myositis (EM) is a specific inflammatory condition of striated muscles, mainly attributable to accumulations of eosinophils [111,124]. It has been found mainly in cattle, occasionally in sheep, and rarely in pigs and horses. The affected animals are usually clinically normal, and EM lesions are discovered at meat inspection after slaughter. Gross lesions consist of green to pale yellow areas that may be up to 15 cm long. The pathogenesis of EM is not clear, and EM lesions have never been found in livestock species experimentally infected with *Sarcocystis* spp [111]. Moreover, the high prevalence of *Sarcocystis* spp infection in naturally infected cattle makes it difficult to designate *Sarcocystis* as the cause of EM. Degenerating sarcocysts are found in sections of lesions of EM [124].

Condemnation of beef containing lesions of EM or grossly visible sarcocysts (*S hirsuta*) can be a serious economic problem [125,126]. In one study, 974 of 1,622,402 (0.06%) cattle slaughtered in 1965 through 1966 in the United States were condemned because of EM [126]. In another report, 18 bovine carcasses from one slaughter plant in the United States were condemned because of grossly visible *S hirsuta* sarcocysts [125].

Diagnosis

The antemortem diagnosis of muscular sarcocystosis can only be made by histologic examination of muscle collected by biopsy [111,127,128]. The finding of immature sarcocysts with metrocytes suggests recently acquired infection, and the finding of mature sarcocysts indicates only past infection [111].

An inflammatory response associated with sarcocysts may help to distinguish an active disease process from an incidental finding of sarcocysts.

Sarcocystis schizonts have not yet been identified in human beings. Although there are several serologic tests and PCR techniques developed experimentally to distinguish *Sarcocystis* species in animals, none have been applied to cases of sarcocystosis in human beings. Tenter [127] has reviewed in detail pitfalls of serologic and molecular diagnosis of sarcocystosis in animals.

The diagnosis of intestinal sarcocystosis is easily made by fecal examination. As has been mentioned, sporocysts or oocysts of sarcocystis are shed fully sporulated in feces, whereas those of *Isospora belli* are often shed unsporulated. It is not possible to distinguish one species of *Sarcocystis* from another by the examination of sporocysts.

Epidemiology and control

Sarcocystis infection is common in many species of animals worldwide [111]. A variety of conditions permit such high prevalence: a host may harbor any of several species of *Sarcocystis*; many definitive hosts are involved in transmission; large numbers of sporocysts may be shed; *Sarcocystis* oocysts and sporocysts develop in the lamina propria and are discharged over a period of many months; oocysts and sporocysts are resistant to freezing and can overwinter on the pasture, or they may be spread by invertebrate transport hosts; there is little or no immunity to reshedding of sporocysts, and each meal of infected meat can thus initiate a new round of sporocyst production; and the fact that *Sarcocystis* oocysts, unlike those of many other species of coccidia, are passed in feces in the infective form frees them from dependence on weather conditions for maturation and infectivity.

Poor hygiene during handling of meat between slaughter and cooking can be a source of *Sarcocystis* infection. In one survey in India, *S suihominis* oocysts were found in feces of 14 of 20 3- to 12-year-old children [121], indicating that meat was consumed raw at least by some, because *S suihominis* can be transmitted to human beings only by the consumption of raw pork. In another study, 3- to 5-year-old children from a slum area were found to consume meat scraps virtually raw, and many pigs from that area harbored *S suihominis* sarcocysts [120]. In European countries, where the frequency of consumption of raw or undercooked meat is relatively high, human beings are likely to have intestinal sarcocystosis. There is no treatment for *Sarcocystis* infection of human beings. On the basis of results in experimental animals, it is probable that sulfonamides and pyrimethamine may be helpful in treating sarcocystosis. There is no vaccine to protect livestock or human beings against sarcocystosis. Shedding of *Sarcocystis* oocysts and sporocysts in feces of the definitive hosts is the key factor in the spread of *Sarcocystis* infection; to interrupt this cycle, carnivores should be excluded from animal houses and from feed, water, and bedding for livestock. Uncooked meat or offal should never be fed to carnivores. Because freezing can drastically reduce or eliminate infectious sarcocysts, meat should be frozen if not cooked.

Exposure to heat at 55°C for 20 minutes kills sarcocysts; thus, only limited cooking or heating is required to kill sporocysts [129]. Dead livestock should be buried or incinerated. Dead animals should never be left in the field for vultures and carnivores to eat.

Summary

In conclusion, much needs to be learned concerning the prevention of *N caninum, T gondii*, and *Sarcocystis* spp infections in livestock. Neosporosis is an enigmatic infection of cattle, and inducing immunity to congenital transfer of *N caninum* is a challenge for immunologists, parasitologists, and veterinarians. Further research is needed regarding the pathogenesis of *N caninum* abortion, the life cycle of the parasite in cattle, and sources of infection. Prevention of transmission of *T gondii* in pregnant women is a major concern. Effects of *Sarcocystis* infections in livestock are difficult to evaluate, because nearly all cattle are infected with *S cruzi*.

References

[1] Dubey JP, Carpenter JL, Speer CA, et al. Newly recognized fatal protozoan disease of dogs. J Am Vet Med Assoc 1988;192:1269–85.
[2] Dubey JP, Barr BC, Barta JR, et al. Redescription of *Neospora caninum* and its differentiation from related coccidia. Int J Parasitol 2002;32:929–46.
[3] Bjerkås I, Mohn SF, Presthus J. Unidentified cyst-forming sporozoon causing encephalomyelitis and myositis in dogs. Z Parasitenk 1984;70:271–4.
[4] Dubey JP, Lindsay DS. A review of *Neospora caninum* and neosporosis. Vet Parasitol 1996; 67:1–59.
[5] Dubey JP. Neosporosis in cattle. J Parasitol 2003;89(Suppl):S42–6.
[6] Dubey JP. Review of *Neospora caninum* and neosporosis in animals. Korean J Parasitol 2003;41:1–16.
[7] Dubey JP, Schares G, Ortega-Mora L. Epidemiology and control of neosporosis and *Neospora caninum*. Clin Microbiol Rev, in press.
[8] McAllister MM, Dubey JP, Lindsay DS, et al. Dogs are definitive hosts of *Neospora caninum*. Int J Parasitol 1998;28:1473–8.
[9] Lindsay DS, Dubey JP, Duncan RB. Confirmation that the dog is a definitive host for *Neospora caninum*. Vet Parasitol 1999;82:327–33.
[10] Gondim LFP, McAllister MM, Pitt WC, et al. Coyotes (*Canis latrans*) are definitive hosts of *Neospora caninum*. Int J Parasitol 2004;34:159–61.
[11] Basso W, Venturini L, Venturini MC, et al. First isolation of *Neospora caninum* from the feces of a naturally infected dog. J Parasitol 2001;87:612–8.
[12] Gondim LFP, Gao L, McAllister MM. Improved production of *Neospora caninum* oocysts, cyclical oral transmission between dogs and cattle, and in vitro isolation from oocysts. J Parasitol 2002;88:1159–63.
[13] Schares G, Pantchev N, Barutzki D, et al. Oocysts of *Neospora caninum, Hammondia heydorni, Toxoplasma gondii* and *Hammondida hammondi* in faeces collected from dogs in Germany. Int J Parasitol 2005;35:1525–37.
[14] Anderson ML, Andrianarivo AG, Conrad PA. Neosporosis in cattle. Anim Reprod Sci 2000;60–61:417–31.

[15] Anderson ML, Reynolds JP, Rowe JD, et al. Evidence of vertical transmission of *Neospora* sp infection in dairy cattle. J Am Vet Med Assoc 1997;210:1169–72.
[16] Dijkstra T. Horizontal and vertical transmission of *Neospora caninum* [PhD dissertation]. Utrecht (The Netherlands): Universiteit Utrecht; 2002.
[17] Ortega-Mora LM, Ferre I, del Pozo I, et al. Detection of *Neospora caninum* in semen of bulls. Vet Parasitol 2003;117:301–8.
[18] Baillargeon P, Fecteau G, Paré J, et al. Evaluation of the embryo transfer procedure proposed by the International Embryo Transfer Society as a method of controlling vertical transmission of *Neospora caninum* in cattle. J Am Vet Med Assoc 2001;218:1803–6.
[19] Davison HC, Guy CS, McGarry JW, et al. Experimental studies on the transmission of *Neospora caninum* between cattle. Res Vet Sci 2001;70:163–8.
[20] Uggla A, Stenlund S, Holmdahl OJM, et al. Oral *Neospora caninum* inoculation of neonatal calves. Int J Parasitol 1998;28:1467–72.
[21] Dijkstra T, Eysker M, Schares G, et al. Dogs shed *Neospora caninum* oocysts after ingestion of naturally infected bovine placenta but not after ingestion of colostrum spiked with *Neospora caninum* tachyzoites. Int J Parasitol 2001;31:747–52.
[22] Thilsted JP, Dubey JP. Neosporosis-like abortions in a herd of dairy cattle. J Vet Diagn Invest 1989;1:205–9.
[23] Anderson ML, Blanchard PC, Barr BC, et al. *Neospora*-like protozoan infection as a major cause of abortion in California dairy cattle. J Am Vet Med Assoc 1991;198:241–4.
[24] Barr BC, Anderson ML, Dubey JP, et al. *Neospora*-like protozoal infections associated with bovine abortions. Vet Pathol 1991;28:110–6.
[25] Anderson ML, Palmer CW, Thurmond MC, et al. Evaluation of abortions in cattle attributable to neosporosis in selected dairy herds in California. J Am Vet Med Assoc 1995;207: 1206–10.
[26] McAllister M, Huffman EM, Hietala SK, et al. Evidence suggesting a point source exposure in an outbreak of bovine abortion due to neosporosis. J Vet Diagn Invest 1996;8:355–7.
[27] McAllister MM, Björkman C, Anderson-Sprecher R, et al. Evidence of point-source exposure to *Neospora caninum* and protective immunity in a herd of beef cows. J Am Vet Med Assoc 2000;217:881–7.
[28] Wouda W. *Neospora* abortion in cattle, aspects of diagnosis and epidemiology [PhD dissertation]. Utrecht (The Netherlands): University of Utrecht; 1998. p. 1–176.
[29] Okeoma CM, Williamson NB, Pomroy WE, et al. Isolation and molecular characterization of *Neospora caninum* in cattle in New Zealand. NZ Vet J 2004;52:364–70.
[30] Sawada M, Kondo H, Tomioka Y, et al. Isolation of *Neospora caninum* from the brain of a naturally infected adult dairy cow. Vet Parasitol 2000;90:247–52.
[31] Okeoma CM, Williamson NB, Pomroy WE, et al. The use of PCR to detect *Neospora caninum* DNA in the blood of naturally infected cows. Vet Parasitol 2004;122:307–15.
[32] Dubey JP, Schares G. Diagnosis of bovine neosporosis. Vet Parasitol 2006;140:1–34.
[33] Dubey JP, Buxton D, Wouda W. Pathogenesis of bovine neosporosis. J Comp Pathol 2006; 134:267–89.
[34] Wouda W, Moen AR, Visser IJR, et al. Bovine fetal neosporosis: a comparison of epizootic and sporadic abortion cases and different age classes with regard to lesion severity and immunohistochemical identification of organisms in brain, heart, and liver. J Vet Diagn Invest 1997;9:180–5.
[35] Álvarez-García G, Collantes-Fernández E, Costas E, et al. Influence of age and purpose for testing on the cut-off selection of serological methods in bovine neosporosis. Vet Res 2003; 34:341–52.
[36] Baszler TV, Gay LJC, Long MT, et al. Detection by PCR of *Neospora caninum* in fetal tissues from spontaneous bovine abortions. J Clin Microbiol 1999;37:4059–64.
[37] Björkman C, Holmdahl OJM, Uggla A. An indirect enzyme-linked immunoassay (ELISA) for demonstration of antibodies to *Neospora caninum* in serum and milk of cattle. Vet Parasitol 1997;68:251–60.

[38] Conrad PA, Sverlow K, Anderson M, et al. Detection of serum antibody responses in cattle with natural or experimental *Neospora* infections. J Vet Diagn Invest 1993;5:572–8.
[39] Dijkstra T, Barkema HW, Eysker M, et al. Evaluation of a single serological screening of dairy herds for *Neospora caninum* antibodies. Vet Parasitol 2003;110:161–9.
[40] Dubey JP, Jenkins MC, Adams DS, et al. Antibody responses of cows during an outbreak of neosporosis evaluated by indirect fluorescent antibody test and different enzyme-linked immunosorbent assays. J Parasitol 1997;83:1063–9.
[41] Jenkins MC, Caver JA, Björkman C, et al. Serological investigation of an outbreak of *Neospora caninum*-associated abortion in a dairy herd in southeastern United States. Vet Parasitol 2000;94:17–26.
[42] Paré J, Hietala SK, Thurmond MC. An enzyme-linked immunosorbent assay (ELISA) for serological diagnosis of *Neospora* sp. infection in cattle. J Vet Diagn Invest 1995;7:352–9.
[43] Schares G, Conraths FJ, Reichel MP. Bovine neosporosis: comparison of serological methods using outbreak sera from a dairy herd in New Zealand. Int J Parasitol 1999;29:1659–67.
[44] Schares G, Bärwald A, Staubach C, et al. Adaptation of a commercial ELISA for the detection of antibodies against *Neospora caninum* in bovine milk. Vet Parasitol 2004;120:55–63.
[45] Björkman C, McAllister MM, Frössling J. Application of the *Neospora caninum* IgG avidity ELISA in assessment of chronic reproductive losses after an outbreak of neosporosis in a herd of beef cattle. J Vet Diagn Invest 2003;15:3–7.
[46] von Blumröder D, Schares G, Norton R, et al. Comparison and standardisation of serological methods for the diagnosis of *Neospora caninum* infection in bovines. Vet Parasitol 2004;120:11–22.
[47] Baszler TV, Knowles DP, Dubey JP, et al. Serological diagnosis of bovine neosporosis by *Neospora caninum* monoclonal antibody-based competitive inhibition enzyme-linked immunosorbent assay. J Clin Microbiol 1996;34:1423–8.
[48] Baszler TV, Adams S, Vander-Schalie J, et al. Validation of a commercially available monoclonal antibody-based competitive-inhibition enzyme-linked immunosorbent assay for detection of serum antibodies to *Neospora caninum* in cattle. J Clin Microbiol 2001;39:3851–7.
[49] Reichel MP, Ellis JT. Control options for *Neospora caninum* infections in cattle—current state of knowledge. NZ Vet J 2002;50:86–92.
[50] Thurmond M, Hietala S. Strategies to control *Neospora* infection in cattle. Bovine Pract 1995;29:60–3.
[51] Dijkstra T, Barkema HW, Hesselink JW, et al. Point source exposure of cattle to *Neospora caninum* consistent with periods of common housing and feeding and related to the introduction of a dog. Vet Parasitol 2002;105:89–98.
[52] Wouda W, Bartels CJM, Dijkstra T. Epidemiology of bovine neosporosis with emphasis on risk factors. Int J Parasitol 2000;30:884–6.
[53] Schares G, Bärwald A, Staubach C, et al. Potential risk factors for bovine *Neospora caninum* infection in Germany are not under the control of the farmers. Parasitology 2004;129:301–9.
[54] Innes EA, Wright SE, Maley S, et al. Protection against vertical transmission in bovine neosporosis. Int J Parasitol 2001;31:1523–34.
[55] Innes EA, Andrianarivo AG, Björkman C, et al. Immune responses to *Neospora caninum* and prospects for vaccination. Trends Parasitol 2002;18:497–504.
[56] Trees AJ, Williams DJL. Endogenous and exogenous transplacental infection in *Neospora caninum* and *Toxoplasma gondii*. Trends Parasitol 2005;21:558–61.
[57] Williams DJL, Trees AJ. Protecting babies: vaccine strategies to prevent foetopathy in *Neospora caninum*-infected cattle. Parasite Immunol 2006;28:61–7.
[58] Barling KS, Lunt DK, Graham SL, et al. Evaluation of an inactivated *Neospora caninum* vaccine in beef feedlot steers. J Am Vet Med Assoc 2003;222:624–7.

[59] Romero JJ, Pérez E, Frankena K. Effect of a killed whole *Neospora caninum* tachyzoite vaccine on the crude abortion rate of Costa Rican dairy cows under field conditions. Vet Parasitol 2004;123:149–59.
[60] Marsh AE, Barr BC, Packham AE, et al. Description of a new *Neospora* species (Protozoa: Apicomplexa: Sarcocystidae). J Parasitol 1998;84:983–91.
[61] Dubey JP, Beattie CP. Toxoplasmosis of animals and man. Boca Raton (FL): CRC Press; 1988.
[62] Frenkel JK, Dubey JP, Miller NL. *Toxoplasma gondii* in cats: fecal stages identified as coccidian oocysts. Science 1970;167:893–6.
[63] Dubey JP, Lindsay DS, Speer CA. Structure of *Toxoplasma gondii* tachyzoites, bradyzoites and sporozoites, and biology and development of tissue cysts. Clin Microbiol Rev 1998;11: 267–99.
[64] Dubey JP, Frenkel JK. Cyst-induced toxoplasmosis in cats. J Protozool 1972;19:155–77.
[65] Speer CA, Dubey JP. Ultrastructural differentiation of *Toxoplasma gondii* schizonts (types B to E) and gamonts in the intestines of cats fed bradyzoites. Int J Parasitol 2005;35: 193–206.
[66] Dubey JP, Frenkel JK. Feline toxoplasmosis from acutely infected mice and the development of *Toxoplasma* cysts. J Protozool 1976;23:537–46.
[67] Dubey JP. Infectivity and pathogenicity of *Toxoplasma gondii* oocysts for cats. J Parasitol 1996;82:957–60.
[68] Dubey JP. Tachyzoite-induced life cycle of *Toxoplasma gondii* in cats. J Parasitol 2002;88: 713–7.
[69] Dubey JP. Unexpected oocyst shedding by cats fed *Toxoplasma gondii* tachyzoites: in vivo stage conversion and strain variation. Vet Parasitol 2005;133:289–98.
[70] Dubey JP. Comparative infectivity of oocysts and bradyzoites of *Toxoplasma gondii* for intermediate (mice) and definitive (cats) hosts. Vet Parasitol 2006;140:69–75.
[71] Dubey JP, Lunney JK, Shen SK, et al. Infectivity of low numbers of *Toxoplasma gondii* oocysts to pigs. J Parasitol 1996;82:438–43.
[72] Dubey JP. Oocyst shedding by cats fed isolated bradyzoites and comparison of infectivity of bradyzoites of the VEG strain *Toxoplasma gondii* to cats and mice. J Parasitol 2001;87: 215–9.
[73] Wallace GD. Serologic and epidemiologic observations on toxoplasmosis on three Pacific atolls. Am J Epidemiol 1969;90:103–11.
[74] Munday B. Serologic evidence for *Toxoplasma* infection in isolated groups of sheep. Res Vet Sci 1972;13:100–2.
[75] Dubey JP, Rollor EA, Smith K, et al. Low seroprevalence of *Toxoplasma gondii* in feral pigs from a remote island lacking cats. J Parasitol 1997;83:839–41.
[76] Kniel KE, Lindsay DS, Sumner SS, et al. Examination of attachment and survival of Toxoplasma gondii oocysts on raspberries and blueberries. J Parasitol 2002;88:790–3.
[77] Frenkel JK, Hassanein KM, Hassanein RS, et al. Transmission of Toxoplasma gondii in Panama City, Panama: a five-year prospective cohort study of children, cats, rodents, birds, and soil. Am J Trop Med Hyg 1995;53:458–68.
[78] Lindsay DS, Dubey JP, Butler JM, et al. Mechanical transmission of *Toxoplasma gondii* oocysts by dogs. Vet Parasitol 1997;73:27–33.
[79] Schares G, Pantchev N, Barutzki D, et al. Oocysts of *Neospora caninum, Hammondia heydorni, Toxoplasma gondii* and *Hammondida hammondi* in faeces collected from dogs in Germany. Int J Parasitol 2005;35:1525–37.
[80] Dubey JP. Toxoplasmosis—a waterborne zoonosis. Vet Parasitol 2004;126:57–72.
[81] Dubey JP, Hill DE, Jones JL, et al. Prevalence of viable *Toxoplasma gondii* in beef, chicken and pork from retail meat stores in the United States: risk assessment to consumers. J Parasitol 2005;91:1082–93.
[82] Dubey JP, Gamble HR, Hill D, et al. High prevalence of viable *Toxoplasma gondii* infection in market weight pigs from a farm in Massachusetts. J Parasitol 2002;88:1234–8.

[83] Bahia-Oliveira LMG, Jones JL, Azevedo-Silva J, et al. Highly endemic, waterborne toxoplasmosis in north Rio de Janeiro State, Brazil. Emerg Infect Dis 2003;9:55–62.
[84] Bowie WR, King AS, Werker DH, et al. Outbreak of toxoplasmosis associated with municipal drinking water. Lancet 1997;350:173–7.
[85] de Moura L, Bahia-Oliveira LMG, Wada MY, et al. Waterborne outbreak of toxoplasmosis, Brazil, from field to gene. Emerg Infect Dis 2006;12:326–9.
[86] Dubey JP, Carpenter JL. Neonatal toxoplasmosis in littermate cats. J Am Vet Med Assoc 1993;203:1546–9.
[87] Dubey JP, Carpenter JL. Histologically confirmed clinical toxoplasmosis in cats—100 cases (1952–1990). J Am Vet Med Assoc 1993;203:1556–66.
[88] Tenter AM, Heckeroth AR, Weiss LM. *Toxoplasma gondii*: from animals to humans. Int J Parasitol 2000;30:1217–58.
[89] Lindsay DS, Dubey JP. Toxoplasmosis in wild and domestic animals. In: Weiss L, Kami K, editors. *Toxoplasma gondii.* The model apicomplexan. Perspective and methods. London: Academic Press; in press.
[90] Dubey JP, Odening K. Toxoplasmosis and related infections. In: Samuel WM, Pybus MJ, Kocan AA, editors. Parasitic diseases of wild mammals. Ames (IA): Iowa State University Press; 2001. p. 478–519.
[91] Dubey JP. A review of toxoplasmosis in wild birds. Vet Parasitol 2002;106:121–53.
[92] Dubey JP, Zarnke R, Thomas NJ, et al. *Toxoplasma gondii, Neospora caninum, Sarcocystis neurona*, and *Sarcocystis canis*-like infections in marine mammals. Vet Parasitol 2003;116: 275–96.
[93] Cole RA, Lindsay DS, Howe DK, et al. Biological and molecular characterizations of *Toxoplasma gondii* strains obtained from southern sea otters (*Enhydra lutris nereis*). J Parasitol 2000;86:526–30.
[94] Lindsay DS, Thomas NJ, Rosypal AC, et al. Dual *Sarcocystis neurona* and *Toxoplasma gondii* infection in a Northern sea otter from Washington State, USA. Vet Parasitol 2001;97:319–27.
[95] Miller MA, Gardner IA, Kreuder C, et al. Coastal freshwater runoff is a risk factor for *Toxoplasma gondii* infection of southern sea otters (*Enhydra lutris nereis*). Int J Parasitol 2002;32:997–1006.
[96] Jones JL, Kruszon-Moran D, Wilson M, et al. *Toxoplasma gondii* infection in the United States: seroprevalence and risk factors. Am J Epidemiol 2001;154:357–65.
[97] Desmonts G, Couvreur J. Congenital toxoplasmosis. A prospective study of 378 pregnancies. N Engl J Med 1974;290:1110–6.
[98] Remington JS, McLeod R, Thulliez P, et al. Toxoplasmosis. In: Remington JS, Klein JO, editors. Infectious diseases of the fetus and newborn infant. Philadelphia: WB Saunders; 2001. p. 205–346.
[99] Luft BJ, Hafner R, Korzun AH, et al. Toxoplasmic encephalitis in patients with the acquired immunodeficiency syndrome. N Engl J Med 1993;329:995–1000.
[100] Dubey JP. Toxoplasmosis. In: Cox FEG, Wakelin D, Gillespie SH, et al, editors. Topley and Wilson's microbiology and microbial infections. Parasitology. London: Hodder Arnold; 2005. p. 422–42.
[101] Dubey JP, Lappin MR. Toxoplasmosis and neosporosis. In: Greene CE, editor. Infectious diseases of the dog and cat. St. Louis (MO): Saunders Elsevier; 2006. p. 754–75.
[102] Lopez A, Dietz VJ, Wilson M, et al. Preventing congenital toxoplasmosis. MMWR Morb Mortal Wkly Rep 2000;49:59–75.
[103] Dubey JP, Kotula AW, Sharar A, et al. Effect of high temperature on infectivity of *Toxoplasma gondii* tissue cysts in pork. J Parasitol 1990;76:201–4.
[104] Kotula AW, Dubey JP, Sharar AK, et al. Effect of freezing on infectivity of *Toxoplasma gondii* tissue cysts in pork. J Food Prot 1991;54:687–90.
[105] Dubey JP, Thayer DW. Killing of different strains of *Toxoplasma gondii* tissue cysts by irradiation under defined conditions. J Parasitol 1994;80:764–7.

[106] Dubey JP, Thayer DW, Speer CA, et al. Effect of gamma irradiation on unsporulated and sporulated *Toxoplasma gondii* oocysts. Int J Parasitol 1998;28:369–75.
[107] Lindsay DS, Collins MV, Jordan CN, et al. Effects of high pressure processing on infectivity of *Toxoplasma gondii* oocysts for mice. J Parasitol 2005;91:699–701.
[108] Lindsay DS, Collins MV, Holliman D, et al. Effects of high-pressure processing on *Toxoplasma gondii* tissue cysts in ground pork. J Parasitol 2006;92:195–6.
[109] Hill DE, Sreekumar C, Gamble HR, et al. Effect of commonly used enhancement solutions on the viability of *Toxoplasma gondii* tissue cysts in pork loin. J Food Prot 2004;67:2230–3.
[110] Buxton D. Toxoplasmosis: the first commercial vaccine. Parasitol Today 1993;9:335–7.
[111] Dubey JP, Speer CA, Fayer R. Sarcocystosis of animals and man. Boca Raton (FL): CRC Press; 1989.
[112] Dubey JP, Lindsay DS, Saville WJA, et al. A review of *Sarcocystis neurona* and equine protozoal myeloencephalitis (EPM). Vet Parasitol 2001;95:89–131.
[113] Dubey JP, Chapman JL, Rosenthal BM, et al. Clinical *Sarcocystis neurona, Toxoplasma gondii*, and *Neospora caninum* infections in dogs. Vet Parasitol 2006;137:36–49.
[114] Dubey JP. Sarcocystosis. In: Cox FEG, Wakelin D, Gillespie SH, et al, editors. Topley and Wilson's microbiology and microbial infections. Parasitology. London: Hodder Arnold; 2005. p. 443–50.
[115] Aryeetey ME, Piekarski G. Serologische *Sarcocystis*-studien an menschen und ratten. Z Parasitenk 1976;50:109–24.
[116] Heydorn AO. Sarkosporidieninfiziertes Fleisch als mögliche Krankheitsursache für den Menschen. Arch Lebensmittelhygiene 1977;28:27–31.
[117] Hiepe F, Hiepe T, Hlinak P, et al. Experimentelle Infektion des Menschen und von Tieraffen (*Cercopithecus callitrichus*) mit Sarkosporidien-Zysten von Rind und Schwein. Arch Exp Vet Med 1979;33:819–30.
[118] Kimmig P, Piekarski G, Heydorn AO. Zur Sarkosporidiose (*Sarcocystis suihominis*) des Menschen (II). Immun Infekt 1979;7:170–7.
[119] Pena HFJ, Ogassawara S, Sinhorini IL. Occurrence of cattle *Sarcocystis* species in raw kibbe from Arabian food establishments in the city of São Paulo, Brazil, and experimental transmission to humans. J Parasitol 2001;87:1459–65.
[120] Solanki PK, Shrivastava HOP, Shah HL. Morphology of sarcocysts of *Sarcocystis miescheriana* (Khun, 1865; Labbe, 1899) and *Sarcocystis suihominis* (Tadros and Laarman, 1976; Heydorn, 1977) from naturally infected domestic pigs (*Sus scrofa domestica*) in India. Indian J Anim Sci 1991;61:1030–3.
[121] Banerjee PS, Bhatia BB, Pandit BA. *Sarcocystis suihominis* infection in human beings in India. J Vet Parasitol 1994;8:57–8.
[122] Beaver PC, Gadgil RK, Morera P. *Sarcocystis* in man: a review and report of five cases. Am J Trop Med Hyg 1979;28:819–44.
[123] Arness MK, Brown JD, Dubey JP, et al. An outbreak of acute eosinophilic myositis attributed to human *Sarcocystis* parasitism. Am J Trop Med Hyg 1999;61:548–53.
[124] Wouda W, Snoep JJ, Dubey JP. Eosinophilic myositis due to *Sarcocystis hominis* in a beef cow. J Comp Pathol, in press.
[125] Dubey JP, Udtujan RM, Cannon L, et al. Condemnation of beef because of *Sarcocystis hirsuta* infection. J Am Vet Med Assoc 1990;196:1095–6.
[126] Imes GD, Migaki G. Eosinophilic myositis in cattle-pathology and incidence. In: Proceedings of the 71st Annual Meeting of the US Livestock Sanitary Association. 1967. p. 111–2.
[127] Tenter AM. Current research on *Sarcocystis* species of domestic animals. Int J Parasitol 1995;25:1311–30.
[128] Markus MB, van der Lugt JJ, Dubey JP. Sarcocystosis. In: Coetzer JAW, Thomson GR, Tustin RC, et al, editors. Infectious diseases of livestock with special reference to Southern Africa. Ni City (South Africa): Oxford University Press Southern Africa; 2004. p. 360–75.
[129] Fayer R. Effects of refrigeration, cooking, and freezing on *Sarcocystis* in beef from retail food stores. Proc Helminthol Soc Wash 1975;42:138–40.

ELSEVIER
SAUNDERS

Vet Clin Food Anim
22 (2006) 673–693

VETERINARY
CLINICS
Food Animal Practice

Ectoparasites of Cattle and Small Ruminants

Roberto Cortinas, DVM[a,*], Carl J. Jones, PhD[b]

[a]*Department of Veterinary and Biomedical Sciences, University of Minnesota, 205 Veterinary Science, 1971 Commonwealth Avenue, St. Paul, MN 55108, USA*

[b]*Department of Entomology and Plant Pathology, 207 Ellington Plant Sciences Building, College of Agricultural Sciences and Natural Resources, University of Tennessee, Knoxville, TN 37996-4560, USA*

Arthropods are among the most numerous creatures on earth, with more than 900,000 species of insects identified [1]. They are successful creatures, occupying nearly all ecosystems and exhibiting a wide variety of behaviors, including parasitizing other multicellular organisms. Though only a few are ectoparasites of humans and animals, the pain, physical damage, reduction in fitness or gain, disease, and economic costs caused by various insects and acarids (ticks and mites) make their control obligatory. In this article, the authors describe the important ectoparasites of livestock and small ruminants in North America.

Understanding the life cycles of these ectoparasites is essential when one is making decisions about their control. Because the life cycles are varied and sometimes complex, details of each are given here. Two different kinds of life cycle are examined. In some instances, the adult arthropod will look very different from a developing immature, as observed in the flies. The change from larva to pupa to adult is referred to as complete metamorphosis (from the Greek word for transformation). By contrast, the change that is observed in some groups (for example, ticks) is gradual in that the immature and mature stages differ only slightly in appearance. This change is called gradual or incomplete metamorphosis.

Integrated pest management (IPM) requires that we use the safest and least invasive control technology available while keeping pest and vector levels below damage thresholds. As in any other war, it is important that we attack the targets when it will cost us the least and help us gain the

* Corresponding author.
E-mail address: cort0004@umn.edu (R. Cortinas).

doi:10.1016/j.cvfa.2006.06.003

most. Some propose that IPM for use in veterinary medicine is different from that used in plant communities because of the mobility of the subjects and the resulting limitations on successful control technology. Additionally, the client generally has become habituated to nearly complete control, rather than simply keeping pest numbers below the economic threshold or vector numbers below the transmission threshold. Nevertheless, use of IPM will often reduce both the financial burden on the client and the cost to the environment.

Arthropods: phylum Arthropoda

Among the common characteristics of arthropods, perhaps the most important is the presence of an exoskeleton with jointed appendages. Briefly, the cuticle of the exoskeleton is impregnated with pigments and sclerotized by means of protein polymerization, creating a tough, protective surface and characteristic color patterns. This protective cuticle with flexible joints defends arthropods against desiccation, lending them the ability to survive in nearly every environment. Other characteristics shared by arthropods include a complete digestive tract, an open circulatory system (hemocoel), separate sexes, eyes (either simple or compound), and a body with observable divisions: head, thorax, and abdomen in insects; capitulum and idiosoma in ticks; and gnathosoma and idiosoma in mites. Although the magic of Hollywood has created some monstrous arthropods for entertainment, the practical weight limit appears to be 22 kg, attained by some lobsters.

Flies: order Diptera

The Diptera, or "true flies," have one pair of wings, although some intimate parasitic species are wingless. Although they all undergo complete metamorphosis, other life-cycle characteristics, including nutritional requirements, parity mode, and larval development sites, vary widely among these insects.

Mosquitoes, black flies, biting midges, and sandflies

Mosquitoes, black flies, biting midges, and sandflies are grouped into the suborder Nematocera. Adults in this group are generally small and delicate, with long, segmented antennae. Females of a few species of this suborder, not including mosquitoes, can complete the first gonotrophic cycle without a blood meal. In general, these ectoparasites may be considered micropredators, because they consume a portion of the host (blood) without killing but do not stay with a single host. As a result, they usually have moderate to broad host specificity.

Mosquitoes are the best known of the blood-sucking insects. The immature stages are found in virtually every aquatic habitat. Adults of various species are active throughout the day, although individual species may only be active for specific periods, such as dawn and dusk. Depending on the species, eggs may be deposited singly or in rafts in sites as diverse as soil, above the waterline of treeholes, or on the water. Eggs may undergo installment hatching or diapause, but once they hatch, the larvae must complete all four larval instars and the pupal stage in water. Both larvae and pupae require air, which they acquire through appendages touching the surface of the water. Surface oils may take advantage of this characteristic to control immatures in small habitats.

Only the females take blood meals, but both male and female adults can be found in nectaries. In most cases the transmission of infectious disease agents by mosquitoes requires two bites, one to acquire the agent from an infected host and a second to transmit it to an uninfected host. At this time, the only mosquito-borne disease that is of concern for ruminant hosts exists only in enzootic foci in Africa (Rift Valley fever). Therefore, the primary effect mosquitoes may have on ruminants is irritation, although Steelman [2] and others have noted the economic effects of unabated mosquito populations on cattle.

Black flies are small dipterans that deposit their eggs in or near running water. Although only 1 to 5 mm in length, these daytime biters can appear in huge swarms, causing severe annoyance and blood loss. Pathogenesis can include toxicosis, dermatitis, allergies, and death (apparently by asphyxiation) in cattle, sheep, and wild ruminants. Black fly fever in humans is a systemic response to black fly salivary antigens, and cattle may have similar symptoms, including nausea and fever. In sheep, the development of pruritic papules in feeding zones has been observed. At least one species serves as a vector for *Onchocerca lienalis* in the United States [3].

The immature stages spend their lives in water. They are filter feeders that remove organic material from the water or actively feed on substrate materials. In temperate climates, there is rarely more than one generation of each species per year, although the succession of species through a summer may make a single species appear to be constantly present. Although eggs typically cannot withstand desiccation, they are the stage at which diapause occurs. As in mosquitoes, females require blood meals and have anesthetic components to their salivary secretions.

Black fly control is generally best practiced when the flies are in their larval habitat or when they are attacking their hosts. With the increasing purity of flowing water in the United States, larval habitat for the black flies has increased. Consequently, more communities are being tormented by black flies and are asking pest and vector control authorities to provide relief. Moderately efficacious control may be provided to livestock operations using pyrethroid pour-ons and other repellent and toxicant compounds.

Culicoides species, or no-see-ums (Ceratopogonidae), are very small flies that deliver no anesthetic when they bite. *Culicoides* vary from 0.6 to 5 mm in length, depending on the species, and often are so small that they penetrate mosquito screening. The female deposits an egg mass after each blood feeding, with the four larval stages growing in moist, often highly organic habitats. It is believed that most species found in temperate regions have only one generation per year.

Generally found less than 500 m from their larval development sites, the adults can serve as vectors for epizootic hemorrhagic disease, a viral wasting disease of deer that is similar to bluetongue disease. Although cattle are the reservoir hosts for bluetongue viruses, the primary hosts are sheep, including bighorn sheep, mule deer, and white-tailed deer. *Culicoides* also serve as the primary vector of *Onchocerca cervicalis*. This nematode is apparently benign in its bovine hosts, although nematodes killed during pest control efforts sometimes cause a severe hypersensitivity that may be alleviated by antihistamines and glucocorticosteroids. Repellent and toxicant compounds often are effective against *Culicoides*, but they require frequent application. As with mosquitoes and black flies, larval habitat modification and treatment are currently the best control strategy.

Adult sand flies (Phlebotominae) resemble mosquitoes, with their long mouthparts, long antennae, and long legs. However, their bodies and wings are hairy, and, during rest, the wings are held approximately 60° from their body. Two species, *Lutzomyia* and *Phlebotomus*, are important vectors of human and animal disease; for North American livestock, several *Lutzomyia* species are notable because they are potential vectors of vesicular stomatitis virus. Adults are weak fliers, generally found on resting places near larval development sites, which may include manure, soil, forest litter, tree holes, nests, burrows, barns, stables, sheds, cellars, cesspools, and other dark, humid sites with organic debris. Females lay several eggs at a time in scattered groups. After 2 to 20 days, small white larvae hatch to feed on decaying organic matter. Larval maturation takes 30 to 60 days, pupation occurs in a week, and adults live from 2 to 6 weeks. Removing organic wastes and feces, sealing cracks and crevices in masonry, limiting the access of the flies to cesspools and similar sites, and other methods of eliminating larval development sites are effective means of control.

Horse flies, deer flies, and snipe flies

Control of horse flies and deer flies (Tabanidae) presents one of the most difficult challenges among ruminant pests. Eggs are oviposited on emergent vegetation in wetlands, and larvae spend nearly 1 year feeding in aquatic or semiaquatic habitats. The larvae move to drier areas for pupation, and the adults emerge as large insects (10 to 30 mm for horse flies and 6 to 10 mm for deer flies). These are stout-bodied flies, often with iridescent sheens on the eyes. Only the female feeds on blood, using an extremely painful bite; the female literally tears through the skin and blood vessels, with mouthparts that act like scissors that are sharpened on both sides. After the fly has completed the meal, the wound often continues to bleed, attracting face flies. Adult tabanids live only a few weeks. Generally, reports of horse fly problems for an entire summer indicate a series of different species emerging at intervals through the season. Both groups prefer shaded pasture areas, but deer flies are often found deeper in the woods.

Most other fly control techniques have been attempted for tabanids, but, unfortunately, they only work under optimal conditions and need constant attention to be successful. Of these, the best results are achieved with pasture management: removing ruminants from marshy pastures, keeping trees to a minimum, draining semiaquatic habitats, and providing small buildings for escape from the flies all yield some success. Chemical controls need frequent application and often do not kill the female until after it has completed its blood meal.

Another painful biter is the snipe fly (*Symphoromyia* spp, Rhagionidae) of the western United States. Although these insects are an annoyance to cattle, bison, deer, and people, they are not known to be disease vectors. The adults are approximately 5 to 15 mm in length with spotted wings. During the summer months, females will swarm hosts in an attempt to feed, because they require a blood meal to complete egg production. Depending on the species, females will oviposit in the moist soils of meadows or grassy woodlands or in decaying vegetation. Larvae are believed to be predators of microfauna.

Muscid flies

The two most common fly pests of ruminant livestock are the house fly and the stable fly. The common house fly, *Musca domestica*, can complete its life cycle in as few as 10 days, and the females, which have a white or light gray abdomen, may deposit as many as 200 eggs in their lifetime. The immature stages (larvae) are called maggots and are most successful in completing their development in moist areas with a high organic content. Moist, decaying manure (in piles or mixed with hay or straw), spilled, moist feed, and ensilage are among their favored habitats. During the final larval stage, the fly may work its way into a drier region where pupation occurs. The barrel-like pupae are immobile and are often prime candidates for biologic control techniques, as discussed later. Male and female house flies feed on almost any available organic matter that they can ingest with their sponging and sucking mouthparts.

House flies can create major problems for livestock operations. Although they do not take blood meals, they can be carriers of a number of important bacterial species, among them *Salmonella* spp and *Escherichia coli* strains (including 0157:H7) [4]. Additionally, frequent concerns are voiced by nonfarming members of the public. Adult house flies can easily move hundreds of yards searching for food and oviposition sites, and, as populations push into rural areas, conflicts between producers and homeowners have escalated into lawsuits and changes in zoning laws [5].

Because of their mobility, house flies are difficult to control as adults. A variety of chemically oriented techniques meet with moderate success, but most tend to be palliative, in that the producer sees dead flies and believes that the overall fly population has been highly affected. Space sprays, baits, and traps all fall into this category. They can be a highly effective part of an integrated control program, but they should not be relied on for the long term or to control severe problems. Probably the single most effective fly control program is sanitation. At the beginning of fly season, sanitation can be especially effective as the larval sites are broken up, removed, and properly treated for fly control. Rather than chemically treating manure piles, it is best to spread manure residue thinly or to compost properly.

Biologic control has been used effectively as a population management technique in confined animal operations. Tiny parasitoid wasps that lay their eggs in fly pupae and cause no damage to vertebrates have proved especially effective in barns, cattle feedlots, and small lots. Because several wasp species are available, it is probably best to check with a livestock extension entomologist to find out which species or combinations of species should be released in a specific region. In conjunction with biologic controls, baits and traps are thought to be both effective and excellent tools for monitoring populations. Use of larvicidal insecticides should be discouraged when biologic controls are being used, because the parasitoids are generally more sensitive to insecticides than are the flies.

Stable flies (*Stomoxys calcitrans*), the second virtually ubiquitous type of pest flies found on ruminants in North America, are sometimes known locally by regional names (dog fly, canoe fly, lawnmower fly). In appearance, the stable fly is approximately the size of a house fly (5 to 7 mm long) but is dark gray with seven spots on the upper (dorsal) surface of the abdomen. It is an obligate micropredator; both sexes take blood meals. The mouthparts of a stable fly project forward when the fly is at rest, giving the appearance of a bayonet. Feeding stable flies slash their way through the skin and blood vessels and feed rapidly on the pool of blood that forms. The life cycle of a stable fly takes nearly 3 weeks under optimum conditions, and the adult female will deposit as many as 400 eggs in her lifetime. Although the larval habitats of the stable fly are similar to those of the house fly, leaning slightly more toward decaying vegetation, the adults require blood meals for mating and feeding and may stay closer to livestock than do house flies. Unfortunately, although the stable fly has traditionally been known as a barnyard pest, recent reports have extended adult habitat to pastures [6]. Increased use of large rolls of hay for storage and feeding has also brought larval development into pastured areas.

Stable flies take two to three blood meals per day, generally feeding on the legs or underside of an animal. Because they do not have an anesthetic in their saliva, they may cause substantial irritation, and foot stomping is a common response. Cattle may also group together, with those in the center being less irritated by flies than those on the outside. During the spring, this behavior has been blamed for the loss of range cattle calves.

Despite the differences in their feeding habits, control technology for the stable fly remains basically the same as that for the house fly. However, the recent tendency of stable flies to attack livestock in pasture, combined with their ability to disperse over greater distances than house flies, may necessitate a search for new and novel methods of control.

Almost exclusively a pest of pastured cattle, the adult horn fly (*Haematobia irritans*) is generally found either on cattle or ovipositing near or under moist cattle manure. Nonetheless, nonbovine hosts are not uncommon; the occasional hungry horn fly will even bite a human. Smaller than stable flies, these dark flies, less than 5 mm long, have the same bayonet-like appearance of the head. Both sexes penetrate the host's skin with their mouthparts to feed on blood, the female feeding as many as 20 or 30 times a day. The flies are generally found on the backs of cattle, though they move to other portions of the body in response to a variety of environmental cues, including excessive heat. Populations on a single animal occasionally number in the thousands, although 100 to 200 flies on a beef cow will cause reductions in the growth rate of her calves. These flies complete their life cycle in 10 to 14 days during the summer and may have many overlapping generations each year.

The continued use of ear tags has caused the development of resistance to a variety of chemicals, including some organophosphates and pyrethroids. Still, tags remain the treatment of choice for most producers. Many other technologies exist for the control of horn flies: walk-through fly traps, which capture the flies as they leave the host, backrubbers, oilers, direct sprays, dust bags, and pour-ons are all available with several chemical agents. Most of these work well. However, it is wise to check the records of clients and provide them with the opportunity to alternate between (for example) organophosphates and pyrethroids each year.

Face flies (*Musca autumnalis*) look similar to house flies, except for the presence of an orange stripe on the abdomen of the female and an orange hue to the abdomen of the male. They normally congregate around the moist openings on any animal, most frequently around the eyes and nostrils, where they feed using their slightly raspy mouthparts. When these mouthparts contact the surface of the bovine eye, they can transmit the causative agent for bovine pink-eye, *Moraxella bovis*, from cow to cow. Although experts debate the importance of the fly's role in maintaining pink-eye in a herd, there is no doubt that they play a part. Face flies may also be seen in a rosette formation surrounding the recent feeding site of a horsefly or other wounds. Face flies deposit their eggs only in fresh bovine manure and are completely dependent on cattle to complete their life cycle, which takes approximately 21 days in the summer. The white pupae are highly calcareous and refractory to most parasitoid oviposition. Although a moderate irritation in the summer, face flies like to overwinter in buildings and may become a major nuisance problem where populations have accumulated.

The primary difficulty in treating adult face flies is their predilection for feeding on the faces of their hosts. This pattern makes it difficult to apply insecticides in all but a few ways. As with the horn fly, success may be achieved with ear tags. Likewise, oilers and backrubbers may be used if the cattle will self-treat. Where feasible, use of feed additives has proved relatively successful when applied over a large area. Because ear tags are generally intended to provide control of both horn flies and face flies, the use of ear tags for face fly control may be limited by resistance in the local horn fly population.

Bottle flies, blow flies, and screwworms

The bottle flies (*Calliphora*, *Lucilia*, *Paralucilia*, *Phaenicia,* and other associated species) and the black blowfly (*Phormia regina*) are strong-flying, shiny metallic flies with similar life cycles. Though associated with carrion, these flies are also responsible for facultative, or secondary, myiasis. Ovipositing females are attracted to decaying animal tissues, as well as infected or necrotic injuries on the skin or mucous membranes of living animals. After hatching, maggots feed on tissue and exudates for a few days to a week, then drop off the host or leave the remains in search of a pupation site. After about a week, pupation is complete and adults emerge. In general, the life cycle is complete in 2 to 4 weeks, depending on ambient temperature. The appearance of these flies after routine procedures (dehorning, castration, and so forth) is a significant animal welfare concern. Indeed, heavy larval infestations have been associated with death. Observation of animals following these procedures and delivery of warranted veterinary care are essential to controlling these ectoparasites. Other control measures include the removal and disposal of aborted fetuses, afterbirths, offal, and carcasses.

The primary screwworm fly (New World screwworm, American screwworm), *Cochliomyia hominivorax*, is of major economic importance and is reportable. Unlike the bottle flies, the screwworm female does not lay eggs on carrion; an abrasion or cut on the skin or mucous membrane is all that is required for the gravid female to lay her eggs. The monandrous (single-mating) female oviposits eggs in batches of 200 to 300 around the dry border of the lesion, whereupon it feeds on the lesion to acquire nutrients for its next gonotrophic cycle. In its lifetime, the prodigious female can lay approximately 3000 eggs. After just 20 hours, maggots hatch and begin to feed on the wound. Over the course of 4 to 10 days, the larvae develop, reaching about 1.5 cm in length on maturation. The maggots then drop from the wound, pupate in the soil for a week, and emerge as adults. The entire life cycle takes approximately 2 to 3 weeks to complete.

As with the bottle flies, common husbandry practices can provide these flies with attractive oviposition sites. Following shearing, dehorning, or castration, animals should be monitored for the development of myiasis, and newborn calves' navels should be dipped to prevent myiasis and secondary infections. However, even simple thorn scratches or tick bites can provide suitable oviposition sites. Timely treatment of infested sites is crucial, because wounds become attractive to other screwworm flies, bottle flies, and blow flies.

The eradication of screwworms in Curacao, Puerto Rico, United States and in most of Mexico and Central America using sterilized males is considered one of the great successes of modern control technology. Today, efforts are aimed at eradicating the fly north of the Panama Canal, as well as on several Caribbean islands. The success of this program may be attributed to many factors, including the diligence of ranchers, the livestock industry, researchers, field personnel, and governmental agencies involved in the project. Biologically, several factors have assisted in making the eradication program a success, but two are noteworthy: First, males are not blood feeders; therefore, the release of massive numbers of sterile males has not been an annoyance. Second, because female screwworm flies mate only once, the likelihood of successful fertilization due to repeated sexual encounters is nonexistent. Additionally, the Screwworm Adult Suppression System has increased the effectiveness of the sterile male technique. The system uses an insecticide combined with a chemical that mimics the scent of animal wounds, thereby attracting and killing gravid females. By using the system before releasing sterile males, one may reduce the density of females and their offspring, thus increasing the impact of sterile male releases in an area.

Bot flies

Although bot flies (Oestridae) generally do not cause severe disease to their specific host, the economic damage incurred by these flies can be significant. Cattle grubs, the larvae of "gad flies" or "heel flies," are found throughout the Northern Hemisphere. The common cattle grub (*Hypoderma lineatum*) is found throughout the United States and Canada, and the northern grub (*H bovis*) is found mainly in Canada and the northern United States. In general, oestrid adults mimic the appearance of bees; *Hypoderma* adults have alternating bands of black and tan with interspersed orange and yellow hairs. The typical hosts are cattle and bison, although small ruminants and horses may occasionally become accidental hosts.

Adult *Hypoderma* are typically active from spring to early summer, although climate may extend or shift the activity period. Gravid females attach their eggs to the hairs of the legs and lower body portions of cattle. Constant attacks by females cause cattle to make panicked dashes ("gadding"), which may result in immediate injury or lowered weight gain during a season of severe fly activity. After 3 to 7 days, grubs hatch from the eggs and penetrate the skin. The larvae spend the next 4 to 6 months migrating in the host's connective tissue. During the winter, common cattle grubs reside next to the esophagus, and northern cattle grubs migrate into the spinal column. At the beginning of spring, the grubs migrate from their resting areas to the dermis of the backline, where they create a warble, a cyst-like structure with a hole where the larva directs its posterior end. As the larvae mature, the warble grows in size, until the bots complete maturation and drop to the ground to pupate. Pupae burrow slightly into the ground and emerge as adults after 1 to 3 months, though the actual duration may vary according to seasonal changes.

During the past 20 years, cattle grub populations and economic losses resulting from them have decreased in North America. The geographic range of *H bovis* has contracted in the United States [7], and economic losses have declined from more than $600 million per year in 1981 to about $66 million in 1987 [8,9]. The introduction of ivermectin in the 1980s was most likely an important reason for the decline, and newer, easy to deliver avermectins may lead to further decreases [7,10]. Sterile male and vaccine technologies may eventually constitute part of an IPM approach to disposal of these parasites [7].

The nasal bot with the most cosmopolitan distribution is *Oestrus ovis* (sheep nasal bot fly). The adult female measures approximately 1 cm, mimics a grayish-brown honeybee, and has vestigial mouthparts. Sheep serve as the primary host for this fly; although goats and llamas can be infested, it is unknown whether they are competent hosts for *Oestrus* [11]. After being placed around and within the nostrils of the host by the female adult, the small (2-mm) first-stage larvae migrate to the mucous membranes of the nasal passages. The larvae attach in the passages for at least 2 weeks under ideal conditions, or as long as 9 months if overwintering, then crawl to the frontal sinuses, where they remain until they mature into third-stage larvae. Once fully developed, the larvae crawl back into the nasal passages, from which they are ejected by sneezing. The larvae enter the soil and pupate into adults. The length of time required for pupation depends on the weather, typically 4 weeks in the summer or the entire winter if pupation occurs in the fall. Unusually heavy infestations can cause inflammation of the mucous membranes with excessive pus formation ("snotty nose").

Deer and other cervids are the primary hosts for the deer nasopharyngeal bot (*Cephenemyia* spp). Severe reactions to this parasite have been noted in llamas [11,12]. The female resembles a honeybee, measuring almost 1.5 cm. The entire life cycles of the five known North American species of *Cephenemyia* are not fully known. The female larviposits either onto the lips or into the nostrils, depending on the species. The first-stage larvae crawl into the nasal cavities, where they remain. After a brief stay, the larvae migrate to the retropharyngeal pouches and develop into fully matured larvae measuring as long as 4 cm. At this time, the larvae are expelled by the host onto the ground, where they pupate and emerge as adult flies after 2 to 3 weeks.

Nasal bots may be controlled with avermectin insecticides. Prediction models may be useful in determining high risk periods, thereby providing the rancher with a tool to limit exposure of susceptible hosts to female flies [13]. By minimizing the sharing of pastures between llamas and wild ungulates, one may reduce the likelihood of *Cephenemyia* pupation sites near llamas and achieve some reduction in infestation [11].

Keds

Commonly confused with a tick, the sheep ked (*Melanophagus ovinus*) is a blood-sucking, wingless fly that is regarded as the most damaging ectoparasite of sheep in North America. The sheep ked is a permanent ectoparasite typically found on the neck, shoulders, abdomen, and thighs. The female lays fully developed larvae that are cemented to the wool. Pupation occurs within a few hours, and after 3 to 4 weeks, depending on temperature, the adults emerge. Mating occurs soon thereafter, though larvae are not deposited for about 2 weeks.

Bites from keds can result in irritation, pruritus, and wool loss. Damage from repeated skin punctures causes hard, firm nodules to develop in sheepskin ("cockle"), reducing its economic value. Reductions in clean, dry weight of fleece, as well as in carcass weights, have been attributed to keds. Producers also blame keds for "back loss," the death of pregnant ewes due to suffocation. In an attempt to scratch, ewes roll on their backs and become stuck, causing the internal organs to press on the diaphragm.

Off the host, keds may survive for a few days, although their longevity is extended when they are insulated in wool, especially under cool and moist conditions. Animal-to-animal contact is probably the most important transmission route, and younger sheep tend to be more heavily infested. Shearing before lambing and subsequently treating with an insecticide can decrease ked burdens in flocks.

Lice: orders Anopleura and Mallophaga

Although taxonomists argue over where and how to divide lice, there is no argument about the existence of two basic kinds of lice. Those that take blood meals by inserting their mouthparts and taking blood from host vessels are called sucking lice or anoplurans. Lice that scrape bits of host skin or feather and ingest strictly that material (except for a few species that may scrape deeply and draw and feed on blood) are called biting lice or mallophagans. All lice are wingless, dorsoventrally flattened insects that are truly parasitic, deriving all of their nutrition for every life stage from their host. They virtually never leave the host, and most die within just a few hours after leaving. Transfer to a new host is almost invariably accomplished by means of host-to-host contact, although a few species have been known to transfer by hitching rides on phoretic insect hosts. This pattern generally occurs with lice that infest avian species.

Lice of ruminants are generally species specific, although pests of bovids may cross to related species, as will some sheep and goat lice (Table 1). Many species are found in specific sites on animals with moderate infestations or on animals enduring infestation with multiple species. For example, the anoplurans on cattle include five species, with two of them, *Solenopotes capillatus* and *Haematopinus quadripertusus*, found almost exclusively on the face and tail, respectively.

In addition to taking blood, the anoplurans cause irritation that results in rubbing, with consequent damage to the haircoat, hide, and wool. Extremely high populations of sucking lice have been implicated in anemia,

phoresy [for-o-see] - A relationship B/w. two species of org. in which the larger (host) transports a smaller (guest).

Table 1
Important North American lice of livestock and small ruminants

Species	Common name	Prinicipal hosts	Affected sites	Geographic distribution
Bovicola (Damalinia) bovis	Cattle-chewing louse, cattle-biting louse	Cattle	Base of tail, shoulders, and top line	Widespread
Bovicola (Damalinia) breviceps	Llama-biting louse	Llama, guanaco, alpaca	Base of tail, sides of neck and body	South America; found on hosts worldwide
Bovicola (Damalinia) caprae	Goat-biting louse	Goats	Base of tail, shoulders, head, neck and back	Widespread
Bovicola (Damalinia) crassipes	Goat-biting louse	Angora goats	Throughout body	Widespread
Bovicola (Damalinia) limbatus	Angora goat–biting louse	Angora goats	Throughout body	Widespread
Bovicola (Damalinia) ovis	Sheep-biting louse	Sheep, bighorn sheep	Back and upper parts	Widespread
Haematopinus eurysternus	Short-nosed cattle louse	Cattle (mature)	Top of neck, brisket, dewlap	Rocky Mountain and Great Plains regions
Haematopinus quadripertusus	Tail switch louse, cattle-tail louse	Cattle	Nymphs: entire body; adults: tail head	Florida, Gulf Coast
Lignonathus africanus	African blue louse	Sheep, goats, mule deer, blacktail deer	Goats: head and neck; other hosts: throughout body	United States, Puerto Rico, Hawaii, Africa, India

Lignonathus ovillus	Face and body louse	Sheep	Summer: face at wool/skin boundary; winter: entire body	Widespread
Lignonathus pedalis	Sheep-foot louse	Sheep	Feet and legs, ventral abdomen, and scrotum	Widespread
Lignonathus stenopsis	Goat-sucking louse	Goats	Throughout body	Widespread
Lignonathus vituli	Long-nosed cattle louse	Calves, dairy cattle	Dewlap and shoulders	Widespread
Microthoracius mazzai		Llama	Head, neck, withers, sides	South America; on hosts worldwide
Microthoracius minor		Llama, vicuña, alpaca	Head, neck, withers, sides	South America; on hosts worldwide
Microthoracius praelongiceps		Llama, guanaco, vicuña	Head, neck, withers, sides	South America; on hosts worldwide
Solenopotes capillatus	Little blue cattle louse	Cattle	Muzzle, dewlap, and neck	Widespread; common in eastern and Gulf Coast United States

abortion, or even death of livestock. In the laboratory, sucking lice can serve as vectors of several diseases to bovines: anaplasmosis, theileriosis, and dermatomycosis. However, it is doubtful that they play a major role in the spread of these diseases.

Because lice are only found on the host, control has proved easy, generally accomplished with a variety of chemical compounds that are applied to the host in the period when lice are most apparent, generally the cool season or winter. In hotter months, louse populations appear to decline and are most likely found on areas of the host where the microclimate is not too hot or dry. Because sucking lice have gut symbionts without which they die, it appears likely that some future control technology will target the symbionts directly.

Mites: orders Prostigmata and Astigmata

More than 250 species of these generally microscopic arthropods cause problems for domestic animals. Only a few have major importance, and the discussion concentrates on those. The most common groups found on ruminants are mites that burrow into the skin of hosts or that penetrate and live in their hair follicles (Table 2). Both groups are obligate parasites that live their lives almost entirely on the host, leaving only to transfer to a new host. Host responses to the presence of mites are the primary reason for concern. The presence of follicle and skin pustular lesions indicates an immune response that may cause the host to scratch until bleeding occurs, frequently resulting in secondary infections. With follicular mites, it is assumed that high populations result from some hormonal cues or from the lack of an appropriate immune response to keep the mites in check.

Creatures like the scabies mites burrow into the outer layers of the host integument, above the stratum granulosum. Female scabies mites burrow through the stratum corneum, creating a tunnel as long as 1 cm that is roughly parallel to the stratum granulosum. The female oviposits two to three eggs per day once she completes her tunneling. Hatched larvae and nymphs make smaller excavations for developmental purposes. Because they are not blood feeders, it appears strange that they should evoke such strong immune responses. However, mite-associated antigens such as feces, cuticular chemicals, and secretions appear at least partially to cause the intense pruritic response to the mites. This response may continue for an extended period, even after successful treatments have been applied. As with many mites, it is difficult to sample for scabies mites. Extensive scrapings down into the stratum granulosum may be required for a positive finding.

Any group of animals in which one scabies-infested host is identified should be treated as if all members are infected. For many years, the most common way to treat infected animals was using dip vats, but the success of new compounds that may be applied as sprays, drenches, and other common techniques has made it both less expensive and less time

Table 2
Important North American mites of livestock and small ruminants

Species	Common name	Hosts	Affected sites	Geographic distribution	Reportable
Chorioptes bovis (caprae, ovis)	Chorioptic mange mite, itchy leg mite, foot mange mite	Cattle, sheep, goats, llamas	Lower legs, scrotum, udder, perineum, tail	Widespread	Yes
Demodex bovis	Cattle follicle mite	Cattle	Withers, neck, back, flanks	Widespread	
Demodex caprae	Goat follicle mite	Goats	Face, neck, shoulders, sides	Widespread	
Demodex ovis	Sheep follicle mite	Sheep	Eyelids, prepuce, vulva	Widespread	
Psorobia (Psorergates) bos (bovis)	Cattle itch mite	Cattle	Neck, brisket, ventral abdomen, body	Australia, United States, Canada, South Africa, Britain	
Psorobia (Psorergates) ovis	Sheep itch mite	Sheep	Entire body	Widespread; eradicated in United States	Yes
Psoroptes aucheniae		Llama	Ears and neck, shoulder, back, tail head	South America; on hosts worldwide	
Psoroptes cuniculi	Rabbit ear mite	White-tailed deer, mule deer, goats, sheep	Sides, brisket, face, ears, base of antlers	On rabbits worldwide	
Psoroptes ovis (bovis)	Scab mite, psoroptic mange mite	Sheep, cattle, goats	Shoulders, rump, entire body	Widespread	Yes
Sarcoptes scabei	Itch mite, sarcoptic mange mite				
var. aucheniae		Llama	Between toes, thighs, axilla, ventrum, perineum, body	South America; on hosts worldwide	
var. bovis		Cattle	Head, neck, shoulders, entire body	On hosts worldwide	Yes
var. ovis		Sheep	Head, face, entire body	On hosts worldwide	Yes

consuming to treat scabies. Again, a key element is the recognition that symptoms may continue after the mites have been eliminated from the host.

Ticks: order Ixodida

Two basic body formations of ticks determine both behavior and the way in which they feed and transmit disease. The Argasidae, or soft ticks, do not have a hard dorsal shield but are covered with a leathery integument that expands far less than the body of a hard tick (Ixodidae). Soft ticks feed for a few minutes many times over their lifespan, increasing their ability to transmit disease to new hosts, and adult females generally have multiple gonotrophic cycles. By contrast, hard ticks have a dorsal protective shield on their abdomen, feed only once during each life stage, and can take from a few days to a week to complete feeding; females invariably undergo a single gonotrophic cycle.

Two soft ticks found in the western United States are of concern to livestock producers. The spinose ear tick (*Otobius megnini*), found in arid and semiarid habitats, is a one-host tick in which the immature stages are obligate blood feeders. Adults have vestigial mouthparts and do not feed, laying their eggs in small batches over a period of as long as 6 months, yet they can survive for as long as 2 years. Adults are found off the host, sheltering in protected niches such as cracks, crevices, and under objects in barns or stables, in which the female lays its eggs. Larvae can survive for as long as 2 months as they seek hosts, and once a host has been located, they crawl to the ear canals to feed. After two feedings and molts, larvae mature into second nymphal instars, which in turn feed and drop off the host to molt into adults. The immature stages feed in the ear canals for 2 to 4 months, causing considerable irritation and pain. Secondary bacterial infections, destruction of the ear canal and tympanic membrane, otitis interna, and even death are possible outcomes. Although it is labor intensive, eradication of protected sites may decrease tick populations. Animal ears should be regularly inspected; if ticks are found, manual removal followed by in situ use of topical insecticides should be considered. Insecticide-impregnated ear tags can control infestation.

The pajaroello tick (*Ornithodoros coriaceus*) occurs along the Pacific Coast, from southern Oregon to Mexico, and is associated with deer or cattle bedding grounds. Besides having a painful "bite," the tick is implicated as the vector of epizootic bovine abortion ("foothill abortion"). Maturation from egg to adult takes about 1 year, and adults generally live for 2 years. After hatching, larvae can live for as long as 5 months while looking for a host. Once successful, they will feed for about 1 week, drop off, and molt into nymphs. The tick molts through seven nymphal instars before it becomes an adult, each molt requiring a blood meal. Nymphs, as well as adults, can live for 2 years without a blood meal. Control of this tick can be difficult because of the short feeding time on the host.

Of the North American hard ticks, the genera *Dermacentor, Ixodes, Amblyomma*, and *Boophilus* are the most important in terms of livestock infestation and disease transmission. The cattle fever tick (*Boophilus annulatus*) and the southern cattle tick (*Boophilus microplus*) are one-host species with similar life cycles. Cattle are the principal hosts, although deer, horses, sheep, and goats may also be infested. After finding a host, larvae mature to the adult stage in about 20 days. The engorged and fertilized female drops off the host to oviposit. After hatching, unfed larvae cannot survive for more than 9 months. Two control techniques contributed to the successful eradication of the tick in the United States: (1) A 2-week acaricidal dipping schedule ensured that recently attached ticks could not complete the 20-day feeding phase. (2) Because livestock were rotated off infested pastures for 9 months, host-seeking larvae died before they could find a host. Intensive surveillance measures at ports of entry are necessary to make certain that these ticks do not re-establish.

Amblyomma species are three host ticks that may feed on large mammals in any of the three feeding stages. They have both eyes and festoons, and females are generally ornate. Their long mouthparts may leave lesions that result in secondary infections when the adult female is finished feeding, or that may simply attract blowflies. *Amblyomma americanum*, the lone star tick, may have a 1- or 2-year life cycle, depending on climate. Originally a southern species, it is believed to have moved as far north as Rhode Island, in conjunction with the recent proliferation of white-tailed deer populations. In the 2-year life cycle, adults are active during the spring, and the resulting larvae emerge in August and overwinter as blood-fed larvae. During the following spring and summer, the nymphs seek blood meals and overwinter. Primarily considered a pest species, causing blood loss and irritation, *A americanum* also plays a role in the transmission of Q fever (*Coxiella burnetti*) and cervid theilerosis (*Theileria cervi*).

Amblyomma maculatum, the Gulf Coast tick, had a historical range of 100 miles or less from the Gulf of Mexico, but it has been an economic pest of cattle as far north as Kansas and Oklahoma for more than 40 years. Larvae and nymphs feed on small rodents and ground-dwelling birds, but the adults have a predilection for the ears of large mammals. Secondary infections, hearing loss, and ear deformities ("gotch ear") are among the problems caused by this species. The tick is capable of serving as a vector for heartwater (*Ehrlichia ruminantium* [=*Cowdria ruminantium*]), which has been found in the Caribbean. Cattle egrets are frequent hosts for the Caribbean vector, *A variegatum*, and there is great concern that a new heartwater focus could develop in the United States with *A maculatum* as the primary vector. Although they have a single-year life cycle, with adults, eggs, larvae, and nymphs appearing in sequential order, its timing differs greatly between southern Texas and Kansas.

The three-host life cycle, in which immature stages feed on small mammals and the adult stage generally seeks large mammals, is typical of most *Dermacentor* species. However, there are two one-host species that infest livestock. The winter tick, *D albipictus*, is found throughout most of the United States and Canada (except Alaska). Its principal hosts are wild ungulates such as moose, deer, and elk, but cattle and horses can also serve as hosts. The life cycle takes approximately 30 days. Larvae begin to search for hosts in the early fall, and ticks are found on hosts from October until March. Though the tick can transmit tick-competent strains of *Anaplasma marginale* [14], a greater problem is the heavy infestations, particularly because the tick is an added burden in the winter, when environmental stresses are high and forage is low. In southern Florida and southern Texas, the tropical horse tick (*D nitens*) typically infests equids, but sheep, goats, cattle, and deer can also serve as hosts. The life cycle takes about 26 days to complete. The tick is typically found in the ears, although in heavier infestations the ticks may be found in the nasal passages, ventral abdomen, and perineum.

The American dog tick (*D variabilis*), Rocky Mountain wood tick (*D andersoni*), and Pacific Coast tick (*D occidentalis*) have typical three-host tick life cycles. The American dog tick is widespread east of the Mississippi River, from Florida and the Gulf Coast states to southeastern Canada, although foci exist in the Pacific Coast, Montana, and Idaho. By contrast, *D andersoni* and *D occidentalis* are found in the western United States. The distribution of the Rocky Mountain wood tick extends from Canada to northern Arizona and New Mexico, and from western Nebraska and South Dakota west through the Rocky Mountains to the Cascade and Sierra Nevada mountain ranges. The distribution of the Pacific Coast tick is more limited; it is typically found in Pacific lowlands from Oregon to California.

In general, immature stages of these ticks feed on small mammals, whereas adults feed on larger mammals. Although adults demonstrate some host preference (*D variabilis* for canids and *D occidentalis* for deer), cattle, sheep, goats, horses, llamas, and humans are suitable hosts. Adult *D occidentalis* may be found year-round, with peak activity in April and May, and nymphs are most abundant during spring and summer. The life cycle of *D andersoni* typically is completed in 1 to 2 years. However, when weather conditions or host availability is poor, it can extend to 3 years, owing to the ability of nymphs and adults to survive as long as a year without a blood meal. Adult *D andersoni* are active in the spring, with populations peaking in April and May. Larval activity generally peaks in July, and nymphs are most active in the spring. The life cycle of *D variabilis* exhibits climatic flexibility across its geographic distribution. In the northern portions of their range, adult *D variabilis* demonstrate two peaks of activity: overwintering adults emerge in the spring, whereas adults appearing later in the summer consist of nymphs that molted during the summer. Peak larval activity occurs in April, and nymphs are more numerous from May to June. In warmer regions, each stage can be active earlier and for an extended period. All three species can cause tick paralysis, as well as transmit *A marginale* and *Francisella tularensis,* the causative bacterium for tularemia. *D andersoni* can transmit the bacterium responsible for Q fever.

Two *Ixodes* species infest livestock in North America: the blacklegged tick ("deer tick"), *I scapularis*, and the western blacklegged tick, *I pacificus*. Immatures of both species primarily feed on small mammals, birds, or reptiles, whereas adults feed on medium and large mammals. *I scapularis* is found in forested habitats in the eastern and central United States and in several provinces in Canada, including Ontario, Manitoba, and possibly Saskatchewan. Though the tick is widely distributed, the greatest foci of activity are in the northeast and north-central United States. The western blacklegged tick parasitizes livestock from Baja California to British Columbia, as well as in a few foci in Nevada, Utah, and Idaho. Both of these ticks transmit *Borrelia burgdorferi,* the agent of Lyme disease, as well as *Anaplasma phagocytophilia,* the agent of granulocytic anaplasmosis.

Effective control of the hard ticks requires knowing when they are likely to be infesting livestock in a particular geographic region. Adults of most three-host species are active during the spring and summer; hence host-targeted acaricide treatments should be used during these periods. Control of one-host ticks can be successful, because all life stages occur on the host and are exposed to any acaricidal treatments. In most cases, a systemic compound with a long period of activity will be most appropriate. Large-scale acaricidal treatment of pastures and other livestock habitats is impractical, expensive, and environmentally unsound. By contrast, habitat modification such as selective grazing and brush control may reduce the risk for tick exposure.

For more than 25 years, scientists have tried to take advantage of host immunity to ticks by developing vaccines against tick antigens. Notable efforts recently have focused on developing vaccines against tick gut antigens, and they have offered hope that vaccines may be developed that will protect against more than one species of tick [15]. In areas of high tick infestation, Asian and African breeds perform much better than their European counterparts, because of their superior ability to become resistant to ixodid ticks after repeated exposures. Biologic control using parasitoids and entomopathogenic fungi has met with limited success. Tick predators are few, but big-headed ants (lion ants, *Pheiodole megacephala*), introduced into the southern United States, the Caribbean, and Hawaii and considered a nuisance species, are exceptional predators [16].

Fire ants: order Hymenoptera

Fire ants are not ectoparasites by any definition of the word. Although they are omnivorous, most pain derives from their sting. Fire ants are excellent at using their sting as a defensive weapon. While grasping with their mandibles, they may sting several times before releasing their grip, rotating on their mandibles. The venom they produce is water insoluble, containing dialkylpiperidine hemolytic factors that induce much of the damage caused by the release of vasoactive amines in mammals.

Along with native fire ant species, we have many other species of ants, some of which help control fire ant populations. However, red imported fire ants, *Solenopsis invicta,* and black imported fire ants, *Solenopsis richteri* (and, where they occur, hybrids of the two species), are considered to be major problems for livestock farms and pastured ruminants in the southern parts of the United States. Damage from fire ants may include damage to machinery from fire ant mounds, seeds and seedling damage, quarantine issues, and human concerns, as well as direct physical damage to ruminants. In a survey [17] of Texas veterinarians, more than 83% of respondents indicated that fire ants could cause economic damage in livestock production. Texas veterinarians reported more than 1200 bovine injuries resulting from fire ant activity. More deaths of bovines, nearly 1400, were reported to have resulted from fire ants. Presumably these deaths are primarily due to the proximity of newborn calves to fire ant mounds, although a causative relationship to fire ant attack is difficult to prove in animals on pasture.

Fire ant control technology is an area that is experiencing tremendous growth, encouraged by the quarantine that many states have placed on movement of agricultural products that can become infested with fire ants. In most situations on farms and ranches, it is important to get the treatment into the nest through the larvae, which chew the food and provide liquid for the adults, including the queen. When one cannot possibly locate every nest in a field, broadcast baits become the control technology of choice. In areas where all nests may be reliably identified, however, it is best to use treatments that will cover individual nests.

References

[1] Eisner T. For the love of insects. Cambridge (MA): Belknap Press of Harvard University Press; 2003.

[2] Steelman CD. Effects of external and internal arthropod parasites on domestic livestock production. Annu Rev Entomol 1976;21:155–78.

[3] Lok JB, Cupp EW, Bernardo MJ, et al. Further studies on the development of *Onchocerca* spp. (Nematoda: Filarioidea) in Nearctic black flies (Diptera: Simuliidae). Am J Trop Med Hyg 1983;32(6):1298–305.

[4] Sasaki T, Kobayashi M, Agui N. Epidemiological potential of excretion and regurgitation by *Musca domestica* (Diptera: Muscidae) in the dissemination of *Escherichia coli* 0157:H7 to food. J Med Entomol 2000;37(6):945–9.

[5] Thomas GD, Skoda SR. Rural flies in the urban environment? Proceedings of a symposium presented at the Annual Meeting of the Entomological Society of America, December, 1989, San Antonio, Texas. Lincoln (NE): Agricultural Research Division, Institute of Agriculture and Natural Resources, University of Nebraska-Lincoln; 1993.

[6] Campbell JB, Skoda SR, Berkabile DR, et al. Research on stable flies and house flies in Nebraska. Nebraska Research Bulletin #341. Lincoln (NE): Agricultural Research Division, Institute of Agriculture and Natural Resources, University of Nebraska-Lincoln; 2001.

[7] Scholl P. Biology and control of cattle grubs. Annu Rev Entomol 1993;38:53–70.
[8] Drummond RO, Lambert G, Smalley HE, et al. Estimated losses of livestock to pests. In: Pimentel D, editor. CRC handbook of pest management in agriculture. Vol. 1. Boca Raton (FL): CRC Press; 1981. p. 111–27.
[9] Drummond RO. Economic aspects of ectoparasites of cattle in North America. In: Leaning WHD, Guerrero J, editors. The economic impact of parasitism in cattle: proceedings of the MSD AGVET Symposium: August 19, 1987, in association with the XXIII World Veterinary Conference, Montreal, Quebec, Canada. Lawrenceville (NJ): Veterinary Learning Systems; 1987. p. 9–24.
[10] Rooney KA, Illyes EF, Sunderland SJ, et al. Efficacy of a pour-on formulation of doramectin against lice, mites, and grubs of cattle. Am J Vet Res 1999;60(4):402–4.
[11] Fowler ME. Medicine and surgery of South American camelids: llama, alpaca, vicuña, guanaco. 2nd edition. Ames (IA): Iowa State University Press; 1998.
[12] Mattoon JS, Gerros TC, Parker JE, et al. Upper airway obstruction in a llama caused by aberrant nasopharyngeal bots (*Cephenemyia* sp.). Vet Radiol Ultrasound 1997;38(5):384–6.
[13] Biggs HC, McClain E, Muller GL, et al. A prediction model for strike in the sheep nasal fly, *Oestrus ovis*, in Namibia. Prev Vet Med 1998;33(1–4):267–82.
[14] Kocan KM, de la Fuente J, Blouin EF, et al. *Anaplasma marginale* (Rickettsiales: Anaplasmataceae): recent advances in defining host pathogen adaptations of a tick-borne rickettsia. Parasitology 2004;129(Suppl):S285–300.
[15] Fragoso H, Rad PH, Ortiz M, et al. Protection against *Boophilus annulatus* populations with the *B. microplus* Bm86-containing vaccine Gavac. Vaccine 1998;16(20):1990–2.
[16] Samish M, Alekseev E. Arthropods as predators of ticks (Ixodoidea). J Med Entomol 2001; 38(1):1–11.
[17] Barr CL, Drees BM. Results from the Texas veterinarian survey: impact of red imported fire ants on animal health. In: Cobb PP, editor. Proceedings of the 1994 Imported Fire Ant Conference, Mobile, Alabama, May 9–11, 1994.

ELSEVIER
SAUNDERS

Vet Clin Food Anim
22 (2006) 695–705

VETERINARY
CLINICS
Food Animal Practice

Diagnostic Methods for Parasitic Infections in Livestock

Lora Rickard Ballweber, MS, DVM*

College of Veterinary Medicine, Mississippi State University, Mississippi State, MS 39762, USA

Parasitic infections are a primary cause of lost productivity in livestock worldwide. Accurate detection of parasites depends on many factors, including collection, storage, and transport of the sample, as well as the method of laboratory evaluation. However, the presence of a particular parasite does not always indicate the presence of parasitic disease. For many parasites, there exists a level at which the effect on production characteristics is balanced by the effect on the development of immunity. Interpretation of test results, therefore, should also consider such factors as the age of the animal or animals, clinical history, nutrition, local epidemiology of the parasites prevalent in the area, and any treatments that have been implemented.

Sample collection

Of necessity, clinical diagnosis of many parasitic diseases is often made by the practitioner without laboratory confirmation. For example, suspected parasitic gastroenteritis often requires treatment before laboratory confirmation becomes available. In other situations, a sharp eye is more valuable than laboratory support, as in the field diagnosis of many ectoparasitic infestations [1,2]. However, when laboratory support is needed or desired, proper choice, collection, and handling of the sample or samples are paramount. Samples should represent the problem that is being investigated and should be taken in sufficient quantity to accurately to perform the test required. The question of how many samples to collect always arises.

* Colorado State University, Department of Microbiology, Immunology, and Pathology, 1619 Campus Delivery, Fort Collins, CO 80523-1619.

E-mail address: lora.ballweber@colostate.edu

doi:10.1016/j.cvfa.2006.06.001 **vetfood.theclinics.com**

This decision depends on the purpose of the investigation and the number of animals involved, among other factors. Although collection of samples from 5% to 10% of the herd is generally given as a rule of thumb [1], it may not be adequate under certain circumstances. For example, fecal egg counts (EPG) can accurately assess the EPG profile of a cattle herd as long as a sufficient number of animals are tested. Fecal EPG values are not normally distributed within a herd; rather, they are overdispersed, with many calves shedding few nematode eggs and a few calves shedding the bulk of the eggs. Consequently, the number of calves tested to assess the EPG profile accurately must include at least one calf from the high-EPG group. Given that the high-EPG group composes an estimated 20% of the herd, a minimum of 15 to 20 animals within the grazing group must be tested to ensure that at least one calf from the high-EPG group is included in the sampling [3].

Fecal samples

Fecal samples are used to detect those parasites inhabiting the gastrointestinal tract, liver, and bile ducts. Parasites inhabiting other parts of the body (eg, lungs) can also be detected using fecal samples when their diagnostic stages pass out of the host by way of the digestive tract. Feces must be fresh, otherwise parasite eggs may develop and larvae hatch. At least 10 g of fresh feces should be collected from the rectum whenever possible; samples picked up from the ground are often contaminated with free-living soil nematodes or fly larvae, which may result in confusion. If samples cannot be examined within 1 to 2 hours, storage at 4°C until examination is recommended. Many parasite stages will remain detectable in feces stored at 4°C for at least 2 months with minimal development. Refrigerated fecal samples may be packed with ice or other coolant and shipped to the laboratory using 24- to 48-hour transport service. Feces should be sent in sealed containers and clearly labeled in indelible marker with the owner's name, animal identification, date of collection, and person responsible for the sample. If samples are pooled, the pen or group identification and number of animals within the group should also be included [4–6].

If feces cannot be cooled, then samples may be stored in 2.5% to 10% formalin. However, such storage can adversely affect the subsequent detection of parasite eggs. Storage by freezing also negatively affects the detection of parasites, whereas storage in 70% ethanol or 100% methanol is unacceptable [7].

Gross examination of feces

The fecal sample should be examined for color, consistency, and the presence of blood, mucus, and grossly visible parasites. In addition, if fecal samples appear old, a notation should be made, because parasite eggs may have hatched and no longer be detectable.

Fecal flotation

The fecal flotation procedure is probably the most commonly used technique for the detection of parasites. It is based on the differences in specific gravity between the parasite's eggs, larvae, cysts, or oocysts and the majority of fecal debris. The specific gravity of most parasite eggs is between 1.1 and 1.2; consequently, specific gravities of the flotation media should be higher than that of the eggs. However, if the specific gravity is too high, more fecal debris will float, concealing the diagnostic stages. Additionally, plasmolysis, osmosis, or rupture of the stages may occur, which can make recognition difficult. Flotation solutions usually have a specific gravity of between 1.2 and 1.3 (Table 1). Flotation media, whether made in-house or commercially available, should always be checked with a hydrometer, which is a simple and inexpensive instrument designed for measuring specific gravity. Several media have been described for use in the flotation procedure, each with advantages and disadvantages. The choice of solution depends on the availability of reagents and the target parasites, although personal preference may also influence the decision [1,4–6]. Many laboratories use saturated sugar solution because (1) less plasmolysis and distortion occur in eggs and oocysts compared with saturated salt solutions; (2) slide preparations from sugar solution may be kept at 4°C for as long as several weeks with a minimum of distortion of eggs; and (3) some parasite eggs float better in sugar solutions [4]. When salt solutions are used, egg distortion occurs within hours, and slides can dry out quickly. The major disadvantage of

Table 1
Preparation and specific gravity of common flotation media

Solution	Specific gravity (approximate)	Formula
Sugar	1.20–1.27	454 g granulated sugar (sucrose)/355 mL tap water; dissolve with gentle heat; once cooled, may add 2–6 mL formaldehyde to deter mold growth
Magnesium sulfate	1.20–1.30	350–450 g $MgSO_4$/1000 mL tap water; gentle heat hastens dissolving
Sodium chloride	1.18–1.20	350–400 g NaCl/1000 mL boiling tap water; conversely, add salt to 1000 mL boiling tap water until the salt no longer dissolves
Zinc sulfate	1.18–1.25	330–386 g $ZnSO_4$/1000 mL tap water; gentle heat hastens dissolving
Sodium nitrate	1.18–1.25	315–400 g $NaNO_3$/1000 mL tap water; gentle heat hastens dissolving

Data from Refs. [4–6,12].

sugar solutions is that they tend to be messy and attractive to flies, ants, and other arthropods.

Qualitative versus quantitative examination

Qualitative fecal examinations simply score the fecal matter according to whether a particular parasite was or was not found. Quantitative fecal examinations provide a count of parasite eggs, usually on a per-gram basis. It is not unusual for grazing ruminants to shed nematode eggs. Consequently, simply finding eggs in an unknown quantity of fecal material gives little valuable information to the practitioner. Quantitative fecal examinations, most often used for gastrointestinal nematodes, provide useful information about pasture contamination, identify animals that repeatedly shed high numbers of eggs, and are essential to evaluating anthelmintic efficacy [2,6]. Several quantitative procedures have been described, but three tend to be the most commonly used. These are the (1) modified double centrifugation technique, (2) modified Stoll egg counting procedure, and (3) McMaster technique. These methods are based on suspension of a known amount of feces in flotation solution. However, the detection limit for each is different, resulting in different levels of precision (Boxes 1 to 3). Choice of technique depends, in part, on expected values. When high egg counts are expected (eg, in many sheep or goat flocks), the McMaster technique is a good choice, whereas it would a poor choice if low egg counts were expected (eg, in adult cattle or in evaluation of anthelmintic resistance).

Fecal sedimentation

The sedimentation technique is primarily used to detect eggs of flukes that do not readily float in the common flotation media. In its most basic form, tap water is combined with feces and the tube allowed to sit briefly undisturbed before the supernatant is decanted (Box 4). This technique allows much of the pigment and lighter debris to be removed, resulting in enhanced visibility of eggs. Centrifugal sedimentation techniques have been described; however, they require organic solvents that need special handling procedures and are unsuitable for use in most veterinary clinics [6]. A commercial apparatus (Flukefinder, Visual Difference Flukefinder, Soda Springs, Idaho), consisting of two sieves, is available in some laboratories specifically for use in the detection of liver flukes eggs. The top sieve removes fecal debris while the bottom sieve retains the fluke eggs. Use of the device cuts the sample preparation time roughly in half.

Baermann technique

The Baermann technique is a method for the extraction of nematode larvae from feces. It is most often used in the detection of lungworm larvae in

Box 1. Modified double centrifugation technique

Homogenize 1–3 g feces in 10–12 mL tap water. Be sure to record weight of fecal material.

Pour mixture through a tea strainer into a beaker. Press the material left behind in the strainer, then discard the material.

Wash the strainer before using again.

Pour contents of beaker into 15-mL centrifuge tube. Fill to top with tap water. If using a fixed-angle rotor, fill tubes to within 1 cm of the top.

Centrifuge the tubes at 300–650× *g* for 5–10 minutes.

Decant the tube and fill one third to one half full with flotation solution. Resuspend the sediment (wooden applicator sticks work well for this). Finish filling with flotation solution.[a]

Place the tube in the centrifuge and add flotation solution by dropper to the tube until a slight inverse meniscus is formed.

Place a 22-mm^2 coverslip on top of the tube. The coverslip should contact the top of the tube without causing the flotation solution to overflow. Centrifuge as before.

Remove the coverslip (lift straight upward) and place on a glass microscope slide. Examine at 100× or higher magnification.

Alternatively, allow the tube to sit undisturbed for 10 minutes before removing the coverslip.

Record count. If original weight of fecal material was >1 g, divide total count by weight of fecal material to obtain eggs per gram.

[a] If using a fixed-angle rotor, add solution to within 1 cm of the top of the tube, then centrifuge as before. After centrifugation, place the tube vertically in a test tube rack, add flotation solution until a slight inverse meniscus is formed, add the coverslip, and allow to stand 10 minutes before removing the coverslip and examining at F100× or higher magnification.

Data from Foreyt WJ. Diagnostic parasitology. In: Veterinary parasitology reference manual. 5th edition. Ames (IA): Iowa State University Press; 2001. p. 3–10; and Dryden MW, Payne PA, Ridley R, et al. Comparison of common fecal flotation techniques for the recovery of parasite eggs and oocysts. Vet Ther 2005;6:15–28.

feces but may also be used to extract larvae from fecal cultures, pasture, soil, or tissues [1,6]. The technique relies on the way warm water stimulates the larvae in the sample to move out of the sample, after which they relax and gravity pulls them to the bottom of the container. Fresh, uncontaminated fecal samples are essential to this procedure (Box 5). Larvae hatching from nematode eggs in aged feces or free-living soil nematodes in

Box 2. Modified Stoll egg counting procedure

Measure 45 mL of tap water into suitable container.
Weigh out 5 g of feces into disposable cup.
Pour some of the water from the container into the cup and mix the feces into a slurry. Transfer the slurry back into the same container the water came from.
Swirl the mixture to create a uniform suspension of the fecal material (do not shake, because this will create unwanted bubbles). The suspension may also be refrigerated for processing later.
Pipette or otherwise remove 1 mL of the suspension into a 15-mL centrifuge tube.
Fill the tube with flotation solution, then place the tube in a centrifuge.
Add flotation solution by dropper to the tube until a slight inverse meniscus is formed. Place a 22-mm^2 coverslip on top of the tube. The coverslip should contact the top of the tube without causing the flotation solution to overflow. Centrifuge at 300–650$\times$ *g* for 5–10 minutes. If using a centrifuge with a fixed-angle rotor, adjust the procedure as described in Box 1.
Remove the coverslip (lift straight upward) and place on a glass microscope slide. Examine at 100$\times$ or higher magnification.
Alternatively, allow the tube to sit undisturbed for 10 minutes before removing the coverslip.
Record count and multiply by 10 to determine eggs per gram.
The math is as follows: 1 mL is 1/50 of the total (45 mL water plus 5 g feces). So 1 mL contains 1/50 of the 5 g of feces, which is 0.1 g of feces examined. 0.1 g feces $\times$ 10 = eggs in 1 g feces.

Data from Hoberg EP, Zimmerman GL, Rickard LG, et al. Efficacy of febantel against naturally acquired gastrointestinal nematodes in calves, and recognition of *Oesophagostomum venulosum* in Oregon cattle. Am J Vet Res 1988;49:1540–2.

contaminated feces may overwhelm the sample and hamper the diagnostician's ability even to find the lungworm larvae.

Blood samples

Since the eradication of babesiosis in the United States, pathogenic hemoprotozoa have been considered uncommon in livestock. Detection of blood parasites has traditionally relied on the examination of Romanowsky-stained blood smears. Using this technique, *Babesia* and *Theileria* are

Box 3. Modified McMaster technique

Homogenize 3 g feces in 15 mL tap water.
Pour mixture through a tea strainer into a beaker. Press the material left behind in the strainer, then discard the material.
Wash the strainer before using again.
Pour contents of beaker into 15-mL centrifuge tube. Centrifuge at 300–650$\times$ *g* for 2 minutes.[a]
Discard supernatant and resuspend sediment in 10 mL flotation solution; decant into a beaker. Add 32 mL additional flotation solution; mix thoroughly.
Using a transfer pipette or syringe, rapidly and gently transfer suspension to one chamber of the McMaster slide. Be careful not to introduce air bubbles into the chamber. Remove fluid and refill the chamber should air bubbles be introduced. Repeat the procedure with the second counting chamber.
Allow to sit undisturbed for 2–4 minutes, then examine both counting chambers. Focusing on the top layer of the solution will result in the grid lines also being in focus. Count only those eggs that are within the grid lines.
Add the counts of the two chambers together and multiply by 50 to obtain eggs per gram. The math is as follows: Each gridded chamber equals 0.15 mL $\times$ two chambers = 0.3 mL examined. 0.3 mL is 1/150 of the total (3 g feces + 42 mL flotation solution). So 0.3 mL contains 1/150 of the 3 g of feces, which is 0.02 g of feces examined. 0.02 g feces $\times$ 50 = eggs in 1 g feces.

[a] Steps 1 to 3 may be omitted and feces mixed directly with the flotation solution. Sugar solutions are not appropriate flotation media for this technique.

Data from Schillhorn van Veen TW. Methods for diagnosis of parasitism in small ruminants. Vet Clin North Am Food Anim Pract 1986;2:335–44; and Foreyt WJ. Diagnostic parasitology. In: Veterinary parasitology reference manual. 5th edition. Ames (IA): Iowa State University Press; 2001. p. 3–10.

visible within the red blood cell. However, the sensitivity of this method is not good, and infections may easily be missed [5]. Detection of other hemoprotozoans, such as *Trypanosoma theileri*, requires culture methods not routinely used in the clinical setting. Although *T theileri* is prevalent in the United States, blood samples are not routinely evaluated for this parasite, because it does require culturing and is not generally recognized as pathogenic [8].

Few serodiagnostic tests that can be incorporated into the clinical setting are commercially available for the detection of ruminant parasites. Test kits are commercially available for *Neospora caninum*, but the procedure

Box 4. Simple fecal sedimentation procedure for detection of fluke eggs

Homogenize 5 g feces in 200 mL tap water.
Pour the mixture through a tea strainer into a beaker. Press the material left behind in the strainer, then discard the material.
Wash the strainer before using again.
Allow the beaker to sit undisturbed for approximately 10 minutes, then decant roughly 70% of the supernatant. Refill the beaker with fresh tap water.
Repeat step 3 until the supernatant is clear (usually three to five times).
Decant 90% of the supernatant and pour the remaining 10% into a Petri dish. A few drops of 0.1% methylene blue dye may be added to the liquid to provide a blue background that contrasts with the yellow fluke eggs that do not stain.
Examine the sediment with a dissecting microscope at 20–30×.

Data from Foreyt WJ. Diagnostic parasitology. In: Veterinary parasitology reference manual. 5th edition. Ames (IA): Iowa State University Press; 2001. p. 3–10.

requires specialized equipment (ELISA plate reader) not usually found in veterinary clinics. However, such equipment is often available in veterinary medical diagnostic laboratories, many of which offer this particular test. Veterinary medical diagnostic laboratories may also be capable of performing serologic testing for other organisms (eg, *Toxoplasma gondii*), and the veterinarian is advised to check with the particular laboratory to find out which services are available.

Ectoparasites

Many ectoparasites are easily recognizable and grossly visible. Others are much smaller, and their presence is determined only after examination of the animal using slight magnification (eg, handheld lens) or microscopic examination of materials collected from the host. However, periodic parasites, which visit the host strictly for a bloodmeal, may not be found on the host at all when evaluated by the clinician.

Examination of hair

Larger ectoparasites (fly larvae, ticks, keds, some lice) may be collected directly from the host using forceps or the end of a moistened paintbrush.

Box 5. Baermann technique for extraction of nematode larvae from feces

Place warm water (approximately 25°C–30°C) into a glass funnel equipped with a wire mesh and stopcock or clamp a rubber hose on the end of the funnel. Fill to just over the wire mesh.
Wrap at least 5 g feces in a piece of double-layer cheesecloth, fully enclosing the feces. Do not crush fecal pellets, because this will result in the fluid's becoming too turbid to examine.
Place the feces on the wire mesh; add additional water to a level of 1–3 cm above the feces.
Allow to sit undisturbed for 6–24 hours. The more feces are present, the longer the apparatus should sit.
Withdraw the bottom 10–15 mL of fluid into a 15-mL centrifuge tube; centrifuge at 300× *g* for 5 minutes.[a]
Pipette the bottom two to three drops from the tube to a microscope slide, add a coverslip, and examine with a compound microscope at 100×.

[a] Straight-sided containers, such as glass jars and beakers, may be preferred. If not using a funnel, remove the fecal sample, then proceed by withdrawing an appropriate amount of liquid from the bottom and placing it into the centrifuge tube.
Data from Refs. [4–6].

Because the mouthparts are important in the identification of ticks, care must be taken to ensure they are not left behind when the tick is removed [9]. As many intact specimens as possible should be collected and placed in sealed containers for subsequent shipment to the diagnostic laboratory. Preservation of specimens in either 70% to 95% ethanol (preferred) or 5% to 10% formalin is desired if samples cannot be shipped soon after collection.

Hairs are collected by brushing, plucking, or both, mounted in mineral oil on a glass slide, and examined microscopically. If collected in the field, they should be transported in a sealed container to ensure that parasites are not lost. Louse eggs, as well as adult lice and some mites, (eg, *Demodex*) may be found by this method [9].

Acetate tape examination

Short strips of acetate tape are repeatedly applied to the hair coat or clipped skin surface to pick up epidermal debris. Surface-dwelling parasites or those living in the coat become attached to the tape, which is then mounted on a glass slide for microscopic examination [5,9]. This technique, often used in companion and exotic animal practices, has not been routinely used for the detection of ectoparasites in livestock, although it is useful for the detection of surface mites.

Skin scraping

Skin scrapings, a routine technique, may be classified into superficial and deep skin scrapes. Superficial skin scrapes, as the name implies, are used to detect surface mites, whereas deep skin scrapes are used for the detection of burrowing and deep follicular mites. In both techniques, multiple scrapings should be taken to maximize the likelihood of detection. Scrapings should be around the edges of active lesions, which is typically where the living mites are found. Clipping the hair before scraping may not be necessary for the superficial skin scrape but is desirable for the deep skin scrape. Clipping before scraping allows for better visualization of the lesion while removing excess hair that can interfere with collection of epidermal debris [5,9].

Scrapings are performed with a blunt scalpel blade or stainless steel spatula. If using a scalpel blade, one must take care to scrape and not cut the skin. Commonly, the blade is dipped in a drop of mineral oil that is on a glass slide, or the drop is placed directly on the skin. For superficial scrapes, only the surface of the skin is scraped. For deep skin scrapes, the skin is squeezed between the thumb and forefinger and scraped until a small amount of capillary blood oozes from the area. After scraping, the emulsion is spread onto the microscope slide, covered with a coverslip, and examined microscopically [5,9]. Skin scrapings may also be performed dry and the material mounted in mineral oil on the slide [9]; however, it may be difficult to transfer the dry material to the slide. Debris from dry skin scrapings may also be digested in 10% potassium hydroxide (20 minutes), followed by centrifugation/flotation to recover the mites.

DNA technology

DNA technology is increasingly being used for the detection of various infectious disease agents. These molecular tools are quite useful in epidemiologic studies; however, there are problems that must be overcome before they become standard diagnostic tools. In many livestock diseases, the high costs and limited availability of the techniques are major issues. The overall usefulness of the technique is also a consideration. Although DNA-based techniques have considerable value in the diagnosis of many viral, bacterial, and protozoal infections, they are not very useful for the diagnosis of gastrointestinal nematode infections [2]. However, a key application of these techniques could be in the early detection of anthelmintic-resistant nematodes, and they could be valuable for exploring the emerging issue of resistance in cattle nematodes.

Quality control and quality assurance

Regardless of the diagnostic tests used, it is the responsibility of the veterinarian to ensure that they are valid and correctly applied. At a minimum, valid tests are ensured through both quality control (steps performed during a test procedure to ensure valid test results) and quality assurance (scheduled, preplanned tasks performed for the same purpose) [10]. Correct application of diagnostic tests involves a basic understanding of the measurements that quantify the value of a test, including false-positive, false-negative, sensitivity, specificity, and positive and negative predictive values [10,11]. The question the veterinarian must ultimately pose, even when using a valid, correctly applied test, is whether the patient will be better off after the test than before.

References

[1] Schillhorn van Veen TW. Methods for diagnosis of parasitism in small ruminants. Vet Clin North Am Food Anim Pract 1986;2:335–44.

[2] Eysker M, Ploeger HW. Value of present diagnostic methods for gastrointestinal nematode infections in ruminants. Parasitology 2000;120:S109–19.

[3] Gasbarre LC, Leighton DA, Bryant D. Reliability of a single fecal egg per gram determination as a measure of individual and herd values for trichostrongyle nematodes of cattle. Am J Vet Res 1996;57:168–71.

[4] Foreyt WJ. Diagnostic parasitology. In: Veterinary parasitology reference manual. 5th edition. Ames (IA): Iowa State University Press; 2001. p. 3–10.

[5] Hendrix CM, Robinson E. Common laboratory procedures for diagnosing parasitism. In: Diagnostic parasitology for veterinary technicians. 3rd edition. St. Louis (MO): Mosby Elsevier; 2006. p. 227–54.

[6] Zajac AM. Fecal examination in the diagnosis of parasitism. In: Sloss MW, Kemp RL, Zajac AM, editors. Veterinary clinical parasitology. 6th edition. Ames (IA): Iowa State University Press; 1994. p. 3–88.

[7] Foreyt WJ. Recovery of nematode eggs and larvae in deer: evaluation of fecal preservation methods. J Am Vet Med Assoc 1986;189:1065–7.

[8] Farrar RG, Klei TR. Prevalence of *Trypanosoma theileri* in Louisiana cattle. J Parasitol 1990;76:734–6.

[9] Wall R, Shearer D. The diagnosis and control of ectoparasite infestation. In: Veterinary ectoparasites: biology, pathology and control. 2nd edition. Oxford (UK): Blackwell Science Ltd.; 2001. p. 179–242.

[10] Wiegers AL. Laboratory quality considerations for veterinary practitioners. J Am Vet Med Assoc 2004;225:1386–90.

[11] Slater MR. Making decisions about diagnostic and screening tests. In: Veterinary epidemiology. St. Louis (MO): Butterworth Heinemann; 2003. p. 71–88.

[12] Dryden MW, Payne PA, Ridley R, et al. Comparison of common fecal flotation techniques for the recovery of parasite eggs and oocysts. Vet Ther 2005;6:15–28.

ELSEVIER
SAUNDERS

Vet Clin Food Anim
22 (2006) 707–712

VETERINARY
CLINICS
Food Animal Practice

Index

Note: Page numbers of article titles are in **boldface** type.

0749-0720/06/$ - see front matter
doi:10.1016/S0749-0720(06)00067-3 *vetfood.theclinics.com*

G

H